To Dale & Colleen,

Blessings and good health to dear friends,

Carol J. Franz

There But For the Grace of God:

Surviving Cancer with Adult Stem Cell Transplants

By Carol J. Franz

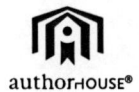
authorHOUSE®

AuthorHouse™
1663 Liberty Drive
Bloomington, IN 47403
www.authorhouse.com
Phone: 1-800-839-8640

© 2009 Carol J. Franz. All rights reserved.

No part of this book may be reproduced, stored in a retrieval system, or transmitted by any means without the written permission of the author.

First published by AuthorHouse 7/7/2009

ISBN: 978-1-4389-6869-8 (sc)
ISBN: 978-1-4389-6870-4 (hc)

Library of Congress Control Number: 2009906176

Printed in the United States of America
Bloomington, Indiana

This book is printed on acid-free paper.

Contents

Acknowledgments vii

Prologue ix

Chapter 1: What's Going On? 1

Chapter 2: What's Up with This Pain? 3

Chapter 3: Uh-Oh, Pain Does Have a Name! 9

Chapter 4: My First Non-Maternity Hospital Stay 11

Chapter 5: Charted Territory 17

Chapter 6: Syracuse, Here I Come 23

Chapter 7: It's Going to be a Long, Long Winter 25

Chapter 8: Spring Brightens my Life 35

Chapter 9: Darkest Moment in the Valley of the Shadow of Death 41

Chapter 10: Hope and Healing 65

Chapter 11: Winter Escape 73

Chapter 12: First Anniversary of my Adult Stem Cell Transplant 75

Chapter 13: Stepping Out 77

Chapter 14: Second Anniversary 85

Chapter 15: Shirts and Letters Tell the Tale 91

Chapter 16: Westward Ho 95

Chapter 17: Still Going Strong 101

Chapter 18: Texas, Here We Come 105

Chapter 19: Election Day in Texas 109

Chapter 20: East is East 113

Chapter 21: Guess What's Back? 119

Chapter 22: Cowboys and Cowgirls 123

Chapter 23: And So it Begins 125

Chapter 24: Letter from the First Lady 127

Chapter 25: Decisions, Treatments and Whatever 129

Chapter 26: Whoops! 139

Chapter 27: Hurry up Already 143

Chapter 28: Here I Go, Ready or Not 145

Chapter 29: Adult Stem Cell Transplant #2 147

Chapter 30: Mission Year 2007 165

Chapter 31: Mrs. Franz Goes to Washington, DC 173

Chapter 32: Jolly Ole England 179

Chapter 33: Busy, Busy and Busier 183

Chapter 34: On the DC Circuit Again -- Is Anyone Listening? 189

Chapter 35: Have Shirts, Will Travel 193

Chapter 36: Carol in the White House, Oh My 195

Chapter 37: President George W. Bush Meets Determined Carol Franz 201

Chapter 38: Home Again But Not for Long 207

Epilogue 211

References and Sources 215

Letters of Encouragement 219

Acknowledgments

Due to the Grace of God I am alive to thank all those whose prayers and care enabled me to share my physically "born again" life through adult stem cell transplants.

I thank my Lord and Savior Jesus Christ.

I also want to thank…

The doctors and nurses who are part of the Lourdes Hospital, Broome Oncology and Syracuse Upstate Medical Hospital transplant teams, Lone Star Oncology, Comprehensive Cancer of Nevada, and finally, Dr. Cooke, Dr. Michaels, and Dr. Fluegel, all of whom are God's instruments.

My husband and primary caregiver, Bill, who cried with me, fed me, encouraged me, nursed me, drove me to endless doctors, treatments and hospitals and brought me Holy Communion.

Kathy Bergmann, who got me settled in at my first hospital stay. Also, she took notes for me when a multiple myeloma survivor talked to me about our cancerous disease. She received flu and pneumonia shots so she would be less likely to expose me to more illness. When I would weakly call out to Bill in our home and he didn't hear me, I'd call Kathy on the phone and then she'd ring back to our house to tell Bill I needed his help. She also helped type and edit my book.

Sarah Hall, who sat quietly with me many times, which gave me comfort knowing someone was in the room, as I drifted in and out of awareness. Many times she drove me to my oncology appointments. She also helped type and edit my book.

Jane Clear who helped edit my book and encouraged me every step of the way.

Karen Bernardo, librarian, author and editor who volunteered to edit my complete manuscript.

Mary Lou Seymour, my wonderful friend from high school, who sat with me almost every evening for three weeks each time I was in the Syracuse transplant room.

Krys Rowell, my Australian mate, who came all those miles from Sydney to encourage me in my battle.

Abigail, my grandchild, who when she was four years old prayed every night that "Grandma would not throw up." The chemo never made me vomit!

Fr. Thomas H. Watts, one of my prayer warriors, who laid hands on me in prayer and informed me that the Lord still had plans for me here on earth.

Bob and Lois Barden who offered to donate their bone marrow to help me.

Diane Fierle who often trimmed my hair at my home to keep me looking my best, helped me get a walker or Zimmer frame, and ran errands for any item I was lacking.

(In December 2005, Diane wrote me saying, "In thinking way back to the beginning of this chapter in your life...I know I questioned many times, 'Dear Lord, why Carol?' when you were diagnosed with multiple myeloma." She added, "I am sure you are finding peace with why" referring to my passion for speaking out on adult stem cell research and its successes, teaching the differences between adult and embryonic research and explaining how only the adult variety has been shown to be successful in helping humans. "You have been an inspiration to me and I love to share your story," Diane concluded. "I am so grateful to have you in my life. Carol Franz, you are amazing.")

Many friends, neighbors and strangers have prayed for me since 2002 for my health and recovery and God's plan for me.

I am so blessed to have all these people and many more in my life.

Prologue

Patty Davis Fitzpatrick said to me, "You are going to write a book."

"Yeah, right," I was thinking. I hadn't attempted to write a book since the 6th grade, when I was in Central School in Owego, New York.

When I saw Patty, I had just gone into the jewelers' for a watchband. I ended up getting prayed over and given the prophetic word that I was to write a book on the adult stem cell transplants that restored my life after I was treated for multiple myeloma cancer. Oh, and my book would also tell of my faith background. I felt overwhelmed but knew if God wanted me to write a book, He'd guide me in all His ways.

My faith background began, as an infant, when I was baptized in the Owego Presbyterian Church. When I was 5 years old, we lived for a year in Apalachin where I attended the Apalachin Methodist Church and the Apalachin Grange meetings with my parents. I still remember the hymns I learned at the Grange. Moving back to Owego, I again attended the Presbyterian Church and their Sunday school classes. I sang in the Children's Choir and as a teenager I taught Sunday school class. Through all this time my faith grew slowly and steadily.

When I married in 1960, I decided to convert to the Roman Catholicism of my husband. I studied the Roman Catholic faith and knew it was another stepping stone for me. As a Catholic woman, I became active teaching First Communion classes, serving as a Eucharistic Minister, joining Marriage Encounter as half of a team couple and guiding teenagers in a Christian Awareness Program. All these activities fueled my faith walk. I grew even more spiritual with a deeper prayer life through the church movements of Cursillo, Life in the Spirit and Charismatic Renewal.

Since the early 70s I have considered myself to be *spiritually* "born again."

So here I go with the story of my being *physically* "born again" by the Grace of God and autologous (self to self) adult stem cell transplants.

Chapter 1: What's Going On?

One day when I helped Mom up off the couch, I experienced my worst shoulder pain ever. I figured I had pulled a muscle and while I was getting some ice for it, Mom was attempting to wash a pair of slacks using half a bottle of detergent -- which sure can make a lot of suds in a washing machine! I wanted to laugh but felt like crying. She was unaware of anything out of the ordinary happening. My life was certainly not what I thought it was going to be in Bill's retirement years from IBM and Lockheed-Martin.

My mother was suffering from Alzheimer's and I wanted to care for her as she had cared for me all my childhood, but physically I didn't feel up to it. Since I was the eldest daughter and lived just one block from my mother, it was obvious to me that I should be her primary caregiver. When I looked at Mom's confused face, I felt love, pity, and sorrow -- and I just longed to help her.

I didn't feel well but I assumed it was due to all the stress caring for Mom and my daughter's divorce. Living in upstate Owego, New York in 2002 shouldn't have been stressful; the village only had 3800 people living in it, and it was a peaceful farming area where the biggest industry was Lockheed-Martin. My three adult children, Craig and his wife Julie, Terry, and Daniel as well as my grandchildren, Tyler, Molly and Abigail were joys to me, and my life wasn't usually this chaotic. But for some reason I was feeling so tired and exhausted that I thought I was a real wimp at 60 years of age.

I kept having recurring, awful headaches to the point where I applied as many as three ice packs at one time in the hope of relieving the pain. I cried uncontrollably because the pain was so severe.

At the time I wasn't up to dealing with Mom, so my husband of 41 years talked with her about the future. She asked Bill to find her a place to live where there were other people her age. I have always kidded around with Bill that "Mom likes you best."

On Mother's Day, I spent the day with Mom, who wanted to use the phone. She said "That damn woman on the phone kept telling me to hang up and dial again." Also Harry, her cat, "wouldn't eat the peanut butter sandwich she made for him" and that upset her. She asked me, "When did the woman say I could move? When is she coming to take me to where I'm going to live?"

She was referring to the social worker who interviewed her about moving. Poor Mom was so confused. It was so scary and frustrating for her. She asked me if she was losing her mind. Every time I was with her, I kissed and hugged her and told her I loved her so she had human touch and contact.

A few days later, Bill, Dan (our son who was visiting us after graduating from the University of Arizona) and I moved Mom, her bedroom set, TV, rocking chair and cat Harry to a boarding house. At the boarding house Mom joined four other elderly women and the family who cared for them. Even though Mom wanted to move and my sister Sue and I agreed, I was getting flack and stress from a few people for putting Mom there. I was feeling pretty depressed until our eldest son, Craig, called to tell us his wife Julie was pregnant again. How exciting to receive cheerful news about another grandchild to love!

Chapter 2: What's Up with This Pain?

A few days later, my chiropractor's assistant said, "Your muscles are a train wreck in your feet, legs, back, and sternum." I assumed it was stress, but there wasn't much I could do about that, since I was receiving daily phone calls from the boarding house due to Mom's erratic behavior. My own symptoms continued to worsen.

In early June, Bill and I drove twenty-one miles to meet with Binghamton General Hospital doctors and two social workers concerning Mom, who was being evaluated at the hospital to determine if she should remain in the boarding house. They wanted her in a nursing home. The doctor just stood there, said very little and then shook Bill's hand as if intending to leave. I wouldn't shake his hand goodbye and told him I wasn't done discussing my mother yet. They were all in a state of shock because I didn't kiss his ring and act like the doctor was a god. I didn't agree with their treatment or what the social workers said about Mom not going back to the boarding house. A nurse at the hospital took me aside later and hinted I should get a second opinion concerning Mom, which I did. Duh! Mom went back to the boarding house.

It didn't help that Mom's extended family undermined my care of her, causing me so much stress and heartache that I couldn't eat, just cry. I went back to the chiropractor due to a pinched nerve and pain in my shoulders and hip. I couldn't even bend over to tie my shoes! I got home to find there had been a mix-up on the medi-van for Mom's transport back to the boarding house. I was laid up and hurting but got the problems solved. I tried swimming and walking in our swimming pool because I thought it would help but it was just too painful.

The summer weather had been so warm and sunny I wanted to be outdoors more. I attempted it but the humidity, which averaged around 80%, drove me back inside the house. I tried doing yoga but my chest hurt and my left arm was numb. I found I had to ice the pain daily. Some folks kept telling me my pain was just arthritis and to ignore it. Another goodie I kept hearing was that I was no "spring chicken" so of course I'd have aches and pains.

A few days later the pain was so incredible that it felt like an elephant was stepping on my chest, so I had Bill drive me to Wilson Hospital's emergency room, about fifteen miles from home. I had chest x-rays, an EKG, and blood work. My right arm had four bruises where a nurse attempted to put an IV line in. All the tests came out fine except for an elevated "sedition" rate, which meant there was infection or inflammation in me. Nonetheless, the doctor told me to go home, rest and take prescription drugs.

Here was a first! I wasn't hungry but had to eat to take the medicine. My chest really ached from armpit to armpit as well as across my back and shoulder blades. I saw both my chiropractor and my family physician and had blood work done. The Emergency Room doctor informed my family physician that I was diagnosed with costochondritis or Tietze Syndrome which would account for the pain in the collarbone and sternum.

I was visiting Mom several times a week but my bones hurt so much I couldn't go as often as I'd have liked. Besides the pain, I had trouble with sinus and allergies. I was getting used to pain every day, but when I tried the ten-minute walk to the center of the village where the shops and post office were, I could only get to the corner of my street before I hobbled back home. For the first time, Bill realized something was terribly wrong since I could hardly walk.

I was and still am a determined woman. Toward the end of the summer, Bill and I went on a previously planned trip to Williamsburg, Yorktown, and Jamestown, Virginia with Craig, Julie and Abbey. I rested a lot, but when we were at Busch Gardens I thought I pulled a muscle in my pelvic area.

Back at home I tried to get an appointment with an arthritis specialist but I had to wait two months. I was still receiving stressful calls as my extended family just didn't understand Alzheimer's disease and questioned my care of my mom. I read all the information I could about Alzheimer's and did everything suggested by the doctor. I loved my mom and of course wanted only what was best for her.

Dr. Cooke, our family physician, called to say my sedition rate still showed problems somewhere in my body. He told me this wasn't normal for a woman my age. He said my sed rate may have been elevated for a long time, possibly even when I lived in England during the late nineties. Dr. Cooke told me to call Dr. Michaels, a rheumatologist, the first thing in the morning and see if a cancellation appointment was available. I was to keep taking Vioxx medicine. There were still no answers on my condition but I did receive paperwork to take to a specialist. Even though I didn't feel well, I cleaned out more of Mom's stuff and gave it to charity. Then I went home as it was getting difficult to walk even though her house was only a block away.

Praise the Lord, I got an appointment with Dr. Michaels at Binghamton General Hospital. He asked lots of questions, checked my eyes, had blood work done and x-rays. I had a bone scan done as well.

In October, Bill and I attended Bill's 45th Owego Free Academy Reunion at the Owego American Legion. I cried when Mary Hinchcliffe (my friend from California) asked me what was wrong as I was "not myself." Susie Dickinson from Owego, New York also questioned me on my health, saying I was too quiet and not dancing or visiting. These women only saw me once in a great while, yet they noticed something wasn't right. Once I got home, my head hurt so badly that I was up until 4 AM.

Three days later I saw Dr. Michaels, who said I had a stress fracture in my pelvis and tendonitis in both shoulders. He sent me for physical therapy and also prescribed pain killers for me. After my visit, Bill drove me straight to a drugstore. I had to walk some distance from where we parked, even though the doctor told both of us I shouldn't walk. Bill was relieved to hear I was not dying and that I had a diagnosis, but he still didn't quite "get" how bad I was feeling.

I was aching something fierce. Bill wanted to go out to eat and at first I said okay, but then I said I was very tired so he parked the car back in the garage and stormed into the house. I went to bed and rested. He wasn't as patient with me since we learned that I wasn't terminal. I've been told it's a "guy thing!" The next day, though, Bill was very helpful. I told him how much I appreciated all he did for me. I kept thinking to myself, what a difference a day makes.

Dr. Cooke put me on medicine for a sinus infection and also showed me a report from Dr. Michaels which said my chest pain was unexplainable. The next day, I saw Dr. Michaels again, who thought my headaches might be giant cell arteritis -- an inflammation which causes the artery to narrow or become blocked, allowing too little blood to pass through. He put me on a high dose of Prednisone. Bill would accompany me to the plastic surgeon for the temporal artery biopsy.

I was still visiting Mom but only two or three times a week, as I felt so exhausted and hurt so much.

Early November, I met with a plastic surgeon, Dr. Peter Fluczk, whose office was near Binghamton General Hospital. Dr. Fluczk made an incision in my head and took a section of artery out for a biopsy. Dr. Fluczk said Dr. Michaels may want the other side done even though there was no pain there. The "glue" used to close the incision near my hairline felt weird and my blonde hair looked a mess. A week later, I went for the other biopsy to be done on the left side artery. Dr. Fluczk said he found only a slight hardening of the arteries. Dr. Michaels said if the new procedure was negative, my Prednisone intake would drop from 60mg to 15mg for about a month, as there was still a 95 sedition rate and inflammation. He took blood for, as he put it, an obscure blood test that he didn't even want to mention, but as none of us knew what caused the 95 sed rate, we would still investigate. (A normal sed rate is around 33.) Bill made a comment suggesting that I was putting on an act about my illness. I replied, "If you are not part of my solution, then you are part of my problem -- and as far as I am concerned, you can just get out of my way."

Prior to Thanksgiving, Bill and I left on a trip to Las Vegas, Nevada to visit our son, Daniel. I blessed his new apartment with holy water.

On November 26, our 42nd wedding anniversary, I started taking 10mg of Prednisone, and put in a call to Dr. Michaels. About 10 PM Pacific Coast Time, Dr. Michaels called me from New York to say I needed to see a hematologist since my blood test showed too much protein was being produced in my blood. He said something that sounded like "benign mono gamma opathy." I told him about the meds, the swelling near my collarbone and on my back at the top of my shoulders, and also that my headaches had returned.

In the early evening, to celebrate our anniversary, Bill and I checked into the Bellagio, a beautiful Italianate hotel and casino. We had dinner at Caesar's Palace and attended the Cirque du Soleil. I soaked in the huge tub in our hotel room, thinking it might help me feel better since I always seem to be aching.

At last the time came for us to return to New York State. Bill was impatient with me as I gimped through the airport. I probably should have used a wheelchair but was hesitant to say so. I slept a great deal on the plane.

When I saw Dr. Cooke, he told me to tell Bill to be patient. Dr. Cooke explained that Bill was mad at the illness as well as his inability to help me get well, which is why it seemed Bill was angry with me. What was it with this guy thing?

Bill and I met again with Dr. Michaels. The doctor wanted to be faxed all information from the hematologist, Dr. Arun Sheth. Dr. Michaels said a blood disorder could be responsible for the muscular and joint pain. Dr. Cooke informed Dr. Michaels he had contacted Dr. Sheth and set up an appointment to meet about my blood work.

I called the home where Mom was and found out she had a cold, so I was unable to visit her.

As we had purchased nonrefundable tickets a while ago, Bill, our friend Kathy and I took a mid-December bus trip to Wellsboro, Pennsylvania Dickens' Festival. The temperature was 19 degrees while we were there. We had a nice day but on the trip home, the pain in my head was the worse it had ever been. I sat in the last seat in the bus so no one would see me and cried most of the two-hour ride home. Kathy told me later that she could hear me and it was obvious I was in great distress.

On December 10, we traveled fifteen miles to Lourdes Hospital to meet with the hematologist. When we entered Dr. Sheth's office I saw that he was also an oncologist and I exclaimed, "Bill, this is a cancer doctor's office!" Dr. Sheth reviewed my bone marrow biopsy, x-rays, and blood tests. He said the blood was producing too much protein and it could be pre-cancer, cancer or none of the above. but in his experience it had never been something else. When I returned home, I telephoned Joan Lewis, my neighbor, who prayed over me. I also called my friend Sarah Hall, who put me on her prayer list and phoned another friend, Sandy Ross, to put me on a prayer chain.

I notified Terry, Craig, Julie and Dan of the tests and Dr. Sheth's suspicions. I also phoned family and friends. It is so wonderful to have a praying community. I received an emotional e-mail from Diane Fierle (see letters of encouragement). My friend Krys called from Australia about the cruise we were planning to do together with our husbands. We'd become very close friends when we lived next door to each other in England. I told her what was going on, and she assured me she'd keep me in her prayers.

I called Darlene, Mom's caregiver at the home, and checked on Mom.

We'd just had a big snow storm, and Bill went outside to clear the snow from our driveway and our neighbors'. He went shopping for groceries but he had to call me several times on his cell phone to find the items on the shelves. Life goes on with everyday occurrences.

I looked up blood disorders on the computer, but it was so discouraging that I thought I'd wait until I had a diagnosis. I had enough trouble; I didn't need to borrow any more!

Chapter 3: Uh-Oh, Pain Does Have a Name!

On December 17, 2002, Bill and I were told by Dr. Sheth that I had cancer --monoclonalgammopathy, a myeloma in the blood marrow. After nine months of searching for answers I had a diagnosis: <u>Stage 2 - Multiple Myeloma</u>. The doctor told us chemo should be started as soon as possible but we could think about it for a week or so. Bill told him we had plans to travel to Malone for Christmas with our son and his family. Dr. Sheth says I could live many more Christmases if I began treatment right away. We decided to start immediately. Statistics say that only 3 out of 100,000 people get this form of cancer. Leave it to me to be unique! It usually affects elderly, black men. HUH!

The first person I called was my hairdresser friend, Diane, and cancelled my hair appointment. Instead, I instead went to a wig shop and chose a blonde pageboy wig. My next stop was to buy a big box of chocolates for myself.

Bill called Craig and told him the news. He called us back a few minutes later and said he was coming home. I told him it wasn't necessary as it is a five-hour car drive for him, but he really wanted to be with me.

We called Dr. Cooke's office on our cell phone and told him about the multiple myeloma cancer diagnosis. Dusty, the receptionist, asked that Bill come into the office alone and I stay in the car. Dr. Cooke talked to Bill about changing roles from husband to caregiver. Dusty sat with me in the car and encouraged me. We contacted Terry and Dan by phone. They wanted to come home but as they both lived so far away, we told them to wait until I had my first chemo treatment and see how I did. We called Krys in Australia and told her we'd have to cancel our cruise plans with them. We called Fr. Watts and all our other friends and relatives to tell them the news. They all encouraged me and said they were praying. I told Mom's caregiver, but as Mom wouldn't understand we didn't say anything to her.

Bill cried a lot and said how strong I was. We both cried at different times but were loving toward each other. I seemed to take the news better than Bill -- he cried every time he looked at me. I was shaken by the diagnosis, but my faith in God gave me strength. I had walked a faith walk all my life and it sustained me.

Chapter 4: My First Non-Maternity Hospital Stay

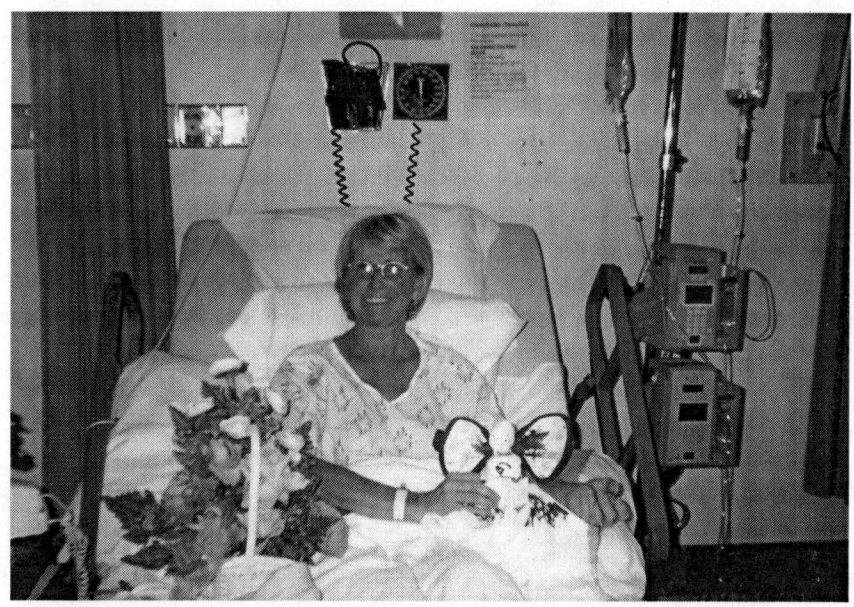

On December 18, Craig, Bill and I went to Lourdes Hospital for my 8 AM appointment in the Oncology Department. A nurse put in a PIC line for treatments at the bend in my left arm. I should have told her I was a lefty and had the PIC line in my right arm. Then I had an x-ray to make sure the line was in correctly. Dr. Sheth talked to Craig, Bill and me before I received my chemo and a saline solution. I had a lunch of turkey sandwich, soup and juice after my treatment. It took a few hours to get a hospital room for me, so Bill and Craig went to visit Mom in the home and took her a box of candy. My pal, Kathy Bergmann, stopped to see me and wound up helping me move to my room. Carmen, my nurse, also got me settled in.

Everyone was so supportive. Nurse Barb Morrissey gave me stones with the words "joy" and "hope" on them. Kathy purchased an angel made out of towels and pot holders to sit on the window sill in my room. That same day, I received silk flowers from my clever relatives Jim & Emy Franz and their sons, Pete and Richie. Peak Performance Physical Therapy sent me a poinsettia arranged with ivy and carnations, but I had to give it away as I couldn't have real flowers due to the spores that might give me an infection. Our daughter Terry called and I spoke to Tyler and Molly as well. Ty and I talked quite a bit. I asked him to pray and go to Mass for G-mama. G-mama is what he called me when he was little and couldn't say Grandma.

I needed all the prayers I could get, because the physical reality of my situation was starting to set in. My face itched, especially my forehead, my eyes felt dry and I had stomach acid/tenderness/burping. The pain killer, Vicodin, that I was given wore off after about five hours. I asked for nausea medicine and received it 45 minutes later.

I shared a room with a very elderly dementia patient who was hard of hearing. She played the TV so loud it could be heard at the end of the hall. In addition, she'd get up and wander about every hour and an alarm would go off. She and the alarm disrupted my rest. Next the bathroom light would go on as she spent about fifteen minutes in the bathroom each time she had to go. I thought I needed to be alone. At 2:30 AM, my nurse Maria and an aide moved me to a new room. They said I should not be exposed to other patients' germs and from then on I'd always have a room to myself.

The next morning, I sat up in a chair and had breakfast. They warmed prune juice in a microwave for me. A therapist took me for a walk and I experienced no hip pain. I got my second bag of chemo and they changed my gown to one with a snap sleeve because I couldn't change gowns with the line that was in my left arm. Lynette came and changed the bandages from the day before.

I found out that Zometa, a bone strengthener, also was given to me intravenously as well as the chemo. I received four days of a chemo mix of Vincristine and Doxorubicin, with Zofran for nausea. I was on a steroid routine of Dexamethansone, 40mg daily, with days on and days off. I took generic Vicodin every six hours for pain. Once a day I took Protonix to help with stomach acid and took Senna-plus -- 2 tablets morning and evening -- to keep stools soft and working. If I did well with chemo for the four days I was in the hospital, my next chemo would be a slow drip done at home -- 96 hours of chemo. At home, I would not be as vulnerable to germs and viruses as I was at the hospital. I was to go to the hospital once a week to get PIC line cleaned and blood taken.

My doctor put me on an antibiotic called Sulfamethoxazole as well as Trimethoprim because I was scheduled to go to Upstate Medical University Hospital in Syracuse to interview for an adult stem cell transplant, and my doctor didn't want me getting any infections that might jeopardize the

There But For the Grace of God

meeting. My appointment at Upstate was my second medical opinion; I believe everyone should get more than one opinion on medical treatments.

In the meantime, though, I felt I was getting into a routine at the hospital, with lots of visitors and encouragement. Craig stopped with a newspaper and e-mails. He told me, "Dad is going to be kinder and more loving as this (meaning the cancer) has woken him up." While Craig was here, Darlene from the chiropractor's office stopped with purple carnations in a vase for me. That made three flower arrangements that I had to give to other patients. Dan called and said I sounded so good that he felt confident I'll be all right. He said, "Dad's crying scared me." Brother James, a chaplain who worked with Fr. Chris at the hospital, stopped to speak to me. Bill arrived and told me he'd received his shots for flu and pneumonia and also told me about all the calls he received at home asking about me. My sister, Sue, called telling me she said a rosary for me every day.

I was in bed ready to go to sleep by 8:30 PM, because every night I was awakened repeatedly for vitals. At 4:30 AM Julie, one of the aides, came to do my vitals and she asked me what cancer I had. We talked briefly. She is one of two survivors of sixteen siblings. After she left, I cried because I wanted to live longer. At 6 AM, when Julie walked past my room, she opened the door when she heard me crying. She held my hand and told me of her sister who survived this cancer. She told me to look in a mirror and tell myself, "I can do all this for I am strong. I will live. I am going to be cured." She encouraged me to focus on flying to visit my children when I got well. She said airlines have an isolated area seating for susceptible flyers but the ticket cost more money than a regular ticket. She made me feel better, and I was able to sleep.

I watched Mass on Channel 6 at 11:30 and communion was brought to me. As the Eucharistic minister licked her fingers while turning pages in a book, I asked her to use her other hand to distribute communion to me. She had me take it by my own hand out of the chalice. People with a healthy immune system are just so unaware of people whose = immune systems are compromised.

In the afternoon Kathy came and stayed for two hours. She gave me Plumeria lotion and bath gel. Diane came for about 1½ hours and brought me candy, a book and a note pad. They were still both there when Joe, who worked with Bill at IBM, stopped to see me and talked about surviving multiple myeloma cancer. He had so much important information that Kathy took notes on the note pad that Diane had just given me. He said, "The family must always speak positively, and the patient must be kept peaceful and positive. Anxiety raises blood pressure and tension makes the pain worse. Focus on keeping mind over matter at all times. Relax the mind, relax the body (which will lessen pain), do slow breathing and picture the word 'remission' written on your forehead." Joe said, whenever friends and family sensed I was down, they should all talk so positively that I would bounce right back. Receiving inspiring cards and notes would help, as does prayer. Family should not get upset or discuss negative things in front of me.

He went on to give me some simple, practical tips. I should be very careful of getting an infection. He suggested my bathroom should be separate from the one used by other family members. As bacteria grow in towels after a couple days, he suggested using paper towels for wiping hands. As Joe spoke, I felt the Lord's presence. I looked at the cross on the wall in my Catholic hospital room and conversed with God, which gave me peace.

Because of the PIC line in my left arm, I began writing with my right, which was no easy task! I hoped I could read my journals that I was keeping through this experience. I have kept a journal ever since Kathy gave me one as a gift to take to Europe. When the chemo tubes were unhooked and I went home, I hoped to write left-handed again.

Kathy called to tell me that her brother-in-law was diagnosed with multiple myeloma, just like me. He was not starting treatment until Monday which was three days away. Brenda Morse called from Colorado to check on me. We have been friends since our kindergarten days and stayed in touch. We have known each other longer than we've known our husbands, which always gave us a chuckle. Bill called and said he had been dusting the house and saw so many memories of our lives together. He was becoming more aware after all these years.

I was so gratified that I had no walking pain. Thank you, Jesus. With Eternal Word Television Network or EWTN on TV, I was able to say a rosary and litany of Jesus and attend Mass.

At last I completed four days of chemotherapy, and I was ready to be discharged! I was given lots of instructions and information. I was told to eat balanced meals. I was to have no vitamins. I was to avoid orange juice and other acid foods that can mess up my stomach. I was to drink lots and lots of water, cranberry juice, and Gatorade so chemo would be flushed through my organs without damaging them. This also helped prevent dehydration and kidney damage. I was to eat no uncooked foods and follow a non-bacterial menu the hospital had me on. I was to avoid caffeine. I was not allowed to eat leftover foods due to the possibility of bacteria in them. I could eat canned foods or processed foods, for example dried fruit. I was to stay away from small children as they carry many germs. No fresh fruits or vegetables, no buffets, and no digging in earth or planting bulbs or seeds for me. When visitors came, I was allowed no hugs or kisses, and I was to sit a safe distance from guests. Dander from animals was to be avoided. As my treatments progressed, I might have to wear a mask to protect myself from infection. I should be careful not to fall. Also I could use nothing on my skin that has alcohol in it. I was not allowed to use scissors or use anything on my nails other than an emery board for fear of getting a cut. I should be careful not to bruise myself. I should get light exercise, just walking slowly in the house, and I was to make sure I lost no weight, especially muscle weight. As Bill was out in the world and I would be pretty much homebound, we decided to use separate bedrooms and separate bathrooms.

As soon as the machines were unplugged and the paperwork was done, I was able to leave. After Bill brought me home from Lourdes Hospital, he prepared lunch for us. I had lots and lots of cards waiting for me. I liked receiving cards, and read them over and over again.

Chapter 5: Charted Territory

My first night home, I hurt a lot so I started Vicodine again, ate prunes and took laxatives so my bowels wouldn't get blocked. I could feel sore spots in my skull where bone was eaten away by the cancer. I took a shower with my arm wrapped in saran wrap to protect the PIC line. Bill made me a pill chart so that there would be no mix-up on my medicine. He was being such a sweetheart and love just glowed from his eyes. He was the man from our early marriage days.

A florist delivered flowers, so I called and explained about my not being able to have flower spores due to the bacteria, but I could receive silk arrangements. They actually took a live plant back and substituted silk! Terry, our daughter, sent me a book called *Hugs* and a lovely letter. (See letters of encouragement)

At 4:30 AM on Christmas Eve Day, I had a muffin and tea, and a few hours later went to the hospital for blood work. I could think of better ways to spend Christmas Eve Day! When we got home, Bill put up the Christmas tree. Craig called and Abbey sang to me. Cathy Franz, my niece from Arizona, visited me and gave me two scarves to cover my head when it got bald. She had been working at Roswell Cancer Research Hospital in Buffalo, New York and told me of survivor cases to encourage me. Sue called to say that St. Paul's Episcopal Church in Owego was praying for me, which gave me great comfort.

On Boxing Day, my nighttime pain pill helped but the pains grew more intense as day went on. I rinsed my mouth as tender spots were developing. My skin was getting really dry and itchy. Bill rubbed lotion on it for me after my shower, but he was so strong I kept telling him to use lighter pressure as he was hurting me. He used my shower and toilet so I had to ask him to please use the other one in the house as Joe had suggested.

I took a steroid pill, which gave me much more energy and less pain. I had hash and eggs for breakfast and a turkey sandwich, cranberry juice and a bowl of chicken noodle soup for lunch. I even did a load of laundry. Also I wrote notes to several people.

Craig called to say Abbey was ill and he took her to the hospital for a strep throat culture. She made a big hit with the hospital staff as she was dressed in her Belle Disney princess gown, heels and accessories that I had given her, Then I talked to Terry, who told me she planned to come up from Duluth, Georgia to spend a long weekend with me in January, which made me very happy.

It had been a good day – but then I went to take a nap about 3:30 PM and woke up screaming. The pain in my chest was a 10 on a scale of 1 to 10. Bill ran in and sat me up. I could breathe short breaths but taking big breaths made my chest hurt like hell. I didn't get much sleep that night. A neighbor plowed her driveway at 11 PM, 1 AM, and 2 AM with her car alarm going off intermittently between 12 AM and 2 AM. I slept from 3 AM on in the recliner in the living room.

In the morning, I called Broome Oncology and Dr. Sheth returned my call. I told him how I couldn't lay down due to the pains in my chest. He said to take more Vicodine and not to do anything strenuous. Dan called so I could hear his voice. He lectured me about allowing Bill to do more to help me.

I continued to receive many calls from friends – one wanted to know when we were coming to stay with friends in London! My friend Mingo called from Bermuda. We met Mingo and her husband Walter when we took a Christian Cruise to Israel, and know we'd always have a place to recuperate whenever we can get to Bermuda. Bill's cousin, Mary Sullivan (Owego, New York) sent me a card saying she was having Masses said for me in Lourdes, France and at The National Shrine of Our Lady of the Snows in Belleville, Illinois. Sue sent me a prayerful card of Jesus. These types of occurrences showed me God is in control.

On my seventeenth day of being cancer-aware, I checked out the International Myeloma Foundation informative site and looked at the shopping places listed there which gave donations to the International Myeloma Foundation when a purchase was made. I registered online with their site, so I would be sent the latest information on multiple myeloma treatments. Bill and I attended Mass at St. John's, Newark Valley. I felt pretty good sitting up and was breathing better. My name was listed for prayer requests along with several other names.

Craig called and told me of the baby shower held for Julie. I had sent a stuffed lamb named Lamb Chop. Abbey informed her mother that the baby can have it when the baby comes to live with them, and Abbey will care of the lamb until then. Thank God my day contained more joy than sadness, as Dr. Sheth said I shouldn't receive any stressful news.

It was getting to be bed time and my chest was hurting a lot. I tried sleeping in the lounge chair again. After an hour, I tried to sleep sitting up on the couch. That wasn't working so then I tried lying on my side in bed. The

There But For the Grace of God

bed worked for two hours, after which I gave up and just sat up in a chair for the rest of the night. My chest was tightening and my breathing shallow. I was hoping my heart was okay.

The next day, my chest still hurt but I was exhausted, so I tried to take a nap. A neighbor's barking dogs kept me awake so I tried a bed upstairs on the other side of the house. I was so tired I was crying. Kathy came over and helped me calm down. She brought me a Miracles calendar and reminded me to believe in miracles. Again, I received many e-mails, phone calls and cards. These helped me get through the day.

On New Year's Eve, my loving, caring husband changed into someone else for a while. Bill had a frustrating time dealing with insurance and pharmaceutical companies over the phone. I used to handle those things before my illness; now he had to handle the stress. The mail from loving people boosted my spirits.

At 8 AM, New Year's Day, Bill fixed me breakfast and brought me my pills. The dogs barking in the neighborhood finished off my sleep. I slept on and off all day. Plus, the constipation was really getting to me! Emy, my niece, visited and brought me canned fruit. She informed me that her son Richie prayed for his Aunt Carol every day. Also, Richie and his cousin Ellen included Aunt Carol in their class prayers at St. Patrick's School as well.

Bill went to see Mom. She "kind of" visited with him, but she was in her own little world. He gave her lots of hugs and she hugged him back.

All my friends named Mary Jane called me that New Year's Day, which has never happened before. I was very tired and finally fell asleep in an actual bed. When I woke at 11 PM, my head was aching big time. I really did have holes in my head (something my dad accused me of as a child), but now they were due to the cancer destroying the bone in my skull. When I awakened at 3 AM soaking wet with sweat, I washed up and got clean pajamas on.

Later that day, we put away the artificial Christmas tree and the ornaments gathered from our many American and foreign trips and special moments in our lives. I wrote an obituary for Mom while my mind was clear enough to do it as I didn't know if she would die before or after me. Bill and I donated money to the Alzheimer Foundation and I put a request for donations to the foundation instead of flowers in Mom's obit as she did not plan to have a public funeral service.

I e-mailed Dan's buddy, Rick Burt, in Tucson, Arizona and received a wonderful e-mail in response to my questions I sent him. Here's his note:

"Hi Carol,

"It was great to hear from you. It sounds like you have quite a road ahead of you with the chemo and steroids. What I told Dan was what I have learned from a few classes I took at the U of A. I'll try to explain as best I can what will be going on with your treatment as I understand it.

"Cells in your body have a normal life cycle. During this cycle, based on the type of cell, the cell will do its intended job inside your body. [For example,] platelets will form a scab if you get cut. White blood cells will attack foreign bodies; red blood cells will carry oxygen to parts of your body.

"During their normal life cycle, cells will also check themselves to make sure that there are no errors in their DNA using 'Check Points.' These 'check points' locate damage or errors and attempt to fix the problem. Cells also have a small part of their life cycle where they reproduce by dividing.

"Most cancers are caused by mutated or confused cells that forget how to do their job. All these mutated cells know how to do is divide. They have lost their ability to fix errors in the DNA and serve no function. They continue to divide uncontrolled. One cell makes two, which then makes four, which then make eight so on and so on. What you are left with is a lump of useless cells or tumor.

"Remember what I said earlier about these cells and their inability to fix errors. Well, each time a cell multiplies more and more errors occur. These errors are then passed to the next generation. It is like how people describe the flu bug. Each year it is different only by a little bit but, after say, five years it barely resembles the original virus. Some of these mutations cause the damaged cells to begin migrating to other parts of the body. These mobile cancer cells are called metastasis or malignant. They invade other tissues and can cause some really serious damage depending on where in your body they decide to plant themselves. It is also much harder to treat malignant cancer because it is throughout your entire body.

"I hope this has explained what cancer is basically. Now how do we fight it?

"Radiation and x-rays are like small bb guns to your cell's DNA. The doctors will shoot holes through all your cell's DNA with x-rays. They do this because normal cells are able to fix the holes with their 'check points.' Cancer cells don't have check points so if their DNA is cut they are unable to fix the holes. The shot-up cancer cells can not reproduce and will die, leaving only the *normal* working cells in your body to reproduce. Chemo works on much the same principal. Damage all cells with specific chemicals and leave only working cells to fix themselves and multiply.

"What is a stem cell? Blood is produced in your bone marrow by special cells. A stem cell is like a blank cell. Its job is to produce new cells. When a stem cell divides it becomes another stem cell as well as a specialized blood cell (red, white, etc.). This process is continuing constantly. The problem is that a stem cell can not divide into two new stem cells. If you lose a stem cell, it is not coming back. (Example: say you have ten stem cells constantly dividing and making new blood cells. In an hour they divide ten times, making a hundred new blood cells, and you still have your ten stem cells. Suddenly one stem cell dies off. You will only produce ninety new blood cells in the next hour. Fewer red blood cells mean fewer cells able to carry oxygen throughout your body causing fatigue. Fewer white blood cells mean fewer police officers inside your body to fight off foreign bodies causing immunosurppression.

"What the doctors are trying to do is take healthy bone marrow with stem cells included and freeze them to keep them alive. Next they are introducing chemo to eradicate all your mutated cells. (Remember cancer cells can not fix themselves but damaged normal cells can.) Once the cancer cells' DNA is shot full of holes and the cells have died, you will be cancer free! Next, new cells from a donor, the frozen ones, will be placed inside your body to replenish your source of stem cells and allow your body to produce new blood cells to give you strength and immunity.

"I hope I explained things well enough so you have a least some idea of what will happen. It is going to be a very tough road. I'm working at the AZ University Medical Center right now and work with the bone marrow transplant patients sometimes. This procedure really wipes them out. They have almost no strength and can barely do anything but sleep. However, their strength and color do come back eventually and it is as if they are reborn with life.

"Remember, don't be afraid to ask questions to your doctor. He is the real expert on the subject. Don't let any doctor intimidate you because he is an MD. You are putting a lot of trust in your doctors; the least they can do is explain what is going on. Don't let any doctor shut up until you are satisfied with the response and has clearly answered your questions.

"My family is praying for you and wishes you and your family the best,

"Rick Burt"

I was so impressed with Rick's response that I passed it on to Kathy, Sue, my kids and others. With my full complement of steroids, pain pills, antibiotics, Senna, etc., I felt pretty good all day and had been busy reading. I slept well for two hours but then my chest and hip started hurting from lying down so I read a complete paperback. At 5:30 AM, I tried to lie down again and sleep.

The next day was a milestone, but not necessarily a happy one. A large clump of my hair came out when I was combing it. This was the first hair loss since I started chemotherapy. I prayed the rosary and attended Mass via the TV. I didn't take phone calls during this time. Bob and Lois Barden, Bill's cousins, offered their bone marrow to me when Bill and I saw them at the drugstore. What a loving gesture but not necessary as I will be using my own adult stem cells for the transplant. A Catholic commented to me that I won't have to spend much time in Purgatory as all my pain and illness will be my Purgatory time here. I was in so much pain, I cried for hours.

Stress on the home front upset me greatly. Joan came over and prayed with me and calmed me down. Bill and I talked about the fact that what he did and said contributed to the stress that made me physically worse. The Parkview Hotel sent me soup for free again, with a note from Joanne saying the soup was a "get well card" from her and her parents.

I received a touching letter from Mike, my high school buddy, and his wife Bette; they were going through cancer treatments with Bette, too. That they took the time to think of me was humbling.

Seven days into January, I'd lost half my hair. I went to Lourdes to get the PIC line cleaned and I was so weak I had to ride in a wheelchair in and out of the hospital. I received lots of cards to boost my spirits. I filled out forms for Upstate Medical in Syracuse for my adult stem cell transplant. Petrina Meyers, a friend, called to pray with me and asked for permission to put me on the Lord Hill Prayer List. Of course, I said yes. I am so blessed to have people praying for me.

Kathy Bergmann had mentioned that her brother-in-law Eric's doctors didn't tell him as much as my doctors told me, so I emailed them some of the information I'd been given on what to avoid with multiple myeloma. I also e-mailed Rick to commend him on his ability to communicate with patients; all my friends who read the letter he sent me thought he would be a wonderful doctor. I dozed off a lot and was sleeping when Ed Mieczkowski left candy and a book for me. I sat on the porch and got some fresh air and sunshine even though it was only 38 degrees outside. That's like summer in January here in Owego.

Another day, I finally got myself dressed but it wasn't easy as I seem to have outgrown some of my clothes, thanks to the steroids. My sweet nephew David called to ask what I'd like him to bring me from Tesco's Super Store in England while he was there. I said, "Cookies with ginger bits in them and some Portmeirion napkins." Joan Meyers Delaney wrote me about the days when Bill and I were her Christian Awareness Program teachers, and how much our being in teenage ministry touched her. She told us that she was now involved with teenagers and their faith growth, and prayed for Bill and me. I needed uplifting things like that to get through this harrowing time.

Chapter 6: Syracuse, Here I Come

Mid-January, I learned that I'd had been accepted into the transplant program and okayed by my insurance. Prior to beginning the procedure, we had to go up for one day for x-rays and a consultation with Dr. Sara Grethlein, whom I really liked. She hugged me goodbye. It helped to have a compassionate, caring doctor, especially in a life or death situation. I'd be in Syracuse for several day trips for cell separation and in the hospital for about three weeks for the transplant and recovery.

Chapter 7: It's Going to be a Long, Long Winter

The next day, we left at 8 AM for Lourdes Hospital and we were there from 9:15 until 2:15. They took blood and hooked me up to the chemo and Zometa solution after that.

We stopped at Penney's and bought two pair of cotton pajamas as mine were all too small now. I was really aching everywhere. The nurses had told me I might have pain from the chemo and Zometa, but by evening I started feeling better.

Craig called at 8:30 to say Olivia Katherine Franz was born on January 15 at 3:45 AM, weighing 7 lbs. 6.8 ounces and measuring 19¾ inches tall. I called relatives to tell them about the baby and of the adult stem cell transplant being approved. Diane stopped at the house and finished cutting off my swatches of hair. Then she took me to the bakery and library in my new wig. Mary McFadden, a young woman from church, stopped at the house. She told me she prayed for me every day and said she couldn't sleep thinking about me. Sometimes she cried at work as she considered me another "Mom." Kathy called and wanted to go to the movies but I was too tired.

I got dressed the next day because of Terry's impending arrival, but I also had other company so it was a good thing I was up and around. Fr. Watts stopped by and Bill fixed us both lunch. After anyone stopped over, Bill always cleaned up with Clorox Wipes so that there were no germs to infect me. Bill left to pick up Terry at the airport, and on their way home they called for directions to the Oreck Vacuum Cleaner Store. Bill had been checking into new vacuums since he started doing the cleaning and realized how poorly our present vacuum worked. Diane helped by purchasing an Oreck and telling us how great it was.

The first day Terry was here, I felt terrible from 4 to 6 AM, with chills, heartburn, and pain. Bill and Terry had lunch at the Parkview, and Joanne sent soup home for me. Dan called to check on his mama and Craig called to say he had set up a website with photographs of the new baby and Abbey. Craig told me that when Abbey got up in the morning she dressed up in her Belle outfit (wig, heels, jewels, dress) because she wanted to show Olivia (who was two days old) what a pretty big sister she had. This made me smile, which was so needed.

The next day, I had my PIC line cleaned and chemo unhooked. This was my first four-day home chemo session with a waist pack. Terry bought Olivia a shirt at the hospital gift shop that said, "I'm the little sister" and I got one for Abbey that said, "I'm the big sister." At home, we all looked at the pictures that Craig had on his website of the baby and her parents and big sister. Terry and Bill attended Mass at St. Patrick's and said everyone at church asked about me. The three of us all cried when I took communion from Bill and Terry. I just sat around reading the Sunday paper while Bill and Terry did all the chores. It was so good having Terry here. I wrapped up in a throw that Mom made as Terry and I visited and laughed. When I rested it was so nice to know that she was just in the other room. It gave Bill a break from care giving, and it was so hard when she finally had to go home.

After taking Terry to the airport, Bill and I headed off for the hospital to see Dr. Sheth. Bill dropped me off in the parking lot and I shuffled into the lobby where I sat and waited for him. When Bill came in, he asked me why I was sitting there instead of going to the doctor's office. I told him I needed someone to hold on to. The tech who took my blood helped me into a wheelchair and took me to the oncology lab where a social worker talked to me. This social worker turned out to have been in my class when I taught aerobics at the Tioga County Boys and Girls Club. I took that as a sign from the Lord as he kept putting people from my past into my life as I went through this struggle. Dr. Sheth said I *must* use a wheelchair and not walk when I came in for treatment as I was too unsteady on my feet.

Because I was having some "female problems," we next went to see Dr. Carol Miller, my OB-GYN. We waited over an hour, for which Dr. Miller apologized. She said that in the future, I should tell the receptionist to inform the doctor immediately that I was there, and she would get me right in. I checked out okay, but she stressed the need for emotional support from people other than just my husband. As it was late in the afternoon, we stopped in a restaurant for lunch. Dr. Sheth said to eat out during off peak hours to avoid crowds. I was now taking Vicodine every four hours to lessen the pain. The doctor assured me I wouldn't become addicted and that every four instead of every six hours was fine.

David Franz stopped at the house and cheered me up with gifts of Botanical Garden Portmeirion linen napkins, the *London Times* and 4 boxes of biscuits with stem ginger. I collected a service for twelve of the Botanical Garden pattern whilst I lived in Burseldon, England as the price was so right there! Terry called as did Donna Bissonnette, an American friend I met in England. My daughter's call was no surprise, but it was humbling to think that so many of the friends I met in England remembered me and wanted to give me encouragement. They didn't realize how they were being "Jesus" to me.

In the morning, I awakened at 6 AM. I was very hungry by 8 AM so I had to wake Bill up to fix me some breakfast. After that Bill left to do grocery shopping and other chores while Sarah visited with me over the telephone. I watched the Right to Life March on C Span TV and listened to President Bush's address. I was still reading the *London Times*. It was my source for a lot of information while living in England. Kathy, God bless her, stopped in with a princess birthday card for me to send to Abbey, as well as items she picked up for me at Arrowhead Christian Bookstore. Later on I really "pigged out" on lollipops for some reason. I wondered if the sub-freezing outdoor temperature and having cabin fever had anything to do with my craving, but I suspect it was the steroids.

That day I overdid it; I felt pretty well at first and after Bill left to run errands, I saw so many chores needing to be done. I wound up fixing my lunch and supper, helping with the laundry and changing my bed linens. The next morning I awoke with new pain under one of my left ribs so I ended up at Lourdes Hospital for x-rays. I met with a doctor filling in for Dr. Sheth while he was on vacation, who prescribed another 14-day round of Vicodin. I had soup for lunch in the hospital canteen and went home to put on one of the lovely new pairs of pajamas my friend Ann Lockwood had purchased for me as a gift. I tended to get so bloated in the night that I had to have larger pair of pj's as all the others were too tight! And I needed warm ones: the nighttime temperature outside was -5 degrees and the wind just kept blowing and blowing.

Not that I spent much time sleeping in my new pajamas! I was up from 2 to 6 AM with severe gas and hardening of my stomach muscles. The agony was so intense that I could barely move. It had been a week since my last chemo and boy, did I hit the wall. Maybe my diet of roast beef, corn, mashed potatoes and an ice cream sundae didn't help. Fortunately, I began to feel a little bit better as the morning went on. Mike Fowler, a friend, called and got me laughing. Dan called to say he was coming east toward the end of July for a golf tournament and to visit his mama. Bill called Jim and Brenda Kelly, some UK friends who were in Clearwater Beach, Florida for a two month vacation. He told them why we wouldn't be down to Florida. Brenda worked for a doctor who was in ten-year remission with multiple myeloma. Of all the Brits to befriend, God paired us up with Brenda and Jim. I needed to hear of survivors like that doctor. What a God-incidence!

Bill went to Mass and I watched Rev. Stanley on TV. Kathy called about going to a movie with her. Dr. Sheth had said I could go to the movies if I went midday when it was not busy. But I was too tired, my head ached, and my nose was bloody.

The following day, I saw Dr. Sheth's substitute. My blood was at 10.3. My kidneys were good. Right then, it was Bill who wasn't up to par; he was having a lot of trouble with muscle spasms that made it hard for him to get around. Barb Morrissey told Bill he was letting down his part of the team by not going to see a doctor when he didn't feel well. He wasn't going to be able to help out with me or do his chores. In other words, go to a doctor!

Bill and I hobbled around trying to get into Target Department Store and we laughed as both of us could barely walk. Fortunately, he could still speak, and later that day I was grateful for his help in dealing with insurance regarding the purchase of a walker (Zimmer frame) for me. And Bill finally consented to see Dr. Cooke about his spasms.

My neighbor, Joan brought me a light and sound machine to block out the dog sounds that kept me awake. But lately, the dog had been less disturbing than my own internal gnarling. I had gas pains big time. I was up in the night for four hours reading, eating crackers and sucking on lollypops. But in the morning, I again felt better; I did two loads of laundry, washed dishes via the dishwasher, made the bed and brought up items stored in the cellar.

Diane called from Wegmann's where she was doing my grocery shopping. When she arrived at the house she unpacked the groceries, shoveled the snow off the sidewalks, picked up lunch for us at Everybody's Country Store and put out the trash bins. What a good friend and helper she was. I stood on the porch and spoke with Avon Conklin, my neighbor, for about 5 minutes. The humidity is 90 percent today and the temperature 20. It seemed really warm!

Sue Ballard visited and brought me a book on angels, a selection of bath and shower soaps, cupcakes and a chicken dinner meal. Sue, an RN, commented how super careful friends had to be preparing food stuffs so that I didn't get an infection. She told me not to worry about being hooked on Vicodin, at least not then. My pain was bad because I'd been trying to stretch the pills out six hours apart instead of four hours. I warmed dinner as Bill slept a great deal due to his medication. Sue's meal was wonderful.

Kathy stopped with a copy of the Sunday *London Times* she bought for me. Wouldn't you know it was missing the section that had the article I wanted to read? I found a pair of jeans I had purchased while in Australia and they fit me. I looked at Spiegel's Catalogue on line and ordered new clothes to lift my spirits. That was definitely a girl thing to do. It also showed that I was planning on sticking around on earth for a while .At 3:30 AM I was finally tired so went to bed. Last thing I read was a morale booster e-mail from Brenda.

I'd only had two hours of sleep the night before so I tried to get more rest. For some reason, Bill had developed a scratchy throat and coughed a lot. I needed to stay away from him. The doctors told him if he ever coughed to pull the neckline of his shirt out and cough down inside his shirt so as not to infect me. He remembered sometimes, but not always. And I couldn't get too upset with him, because he was really a mess. He went to the chiropractor, took some painkillers and then slept. His muscles were still in spasm and he could barely move. We looked comical trying to get around the house. Joan Lewis picked up stuff for me at the drugstore and shopped at Sam's Club in Vestal for me. Good news, though: we heard from our insurance company that I received permission for a walker.

Sarah took me to the hospital to give Bill a break and then we went to the Arrowhead Christian Store in Johnson City and also the Catholic Shop. I felt "normal" but my clothes were uncomfortable. Those steroids really pumped me up.

Lynette from Oncology called, and told me not to take any more steroids until February 11. Terry called too, and I felt led to pray for her ex that the Lord touch his heart and reside there, and that all those I pray for invite Jesus to become Lord of their lives in the name of Jesus.

At 1:30 AM Krys called from Sidney, Australia. She was coming to United States to visit her sister who was temporarily residing in Virginia. She said she'd come to Owego for about a week to visit me and help out with caregiving. Judy Riesbeck took me to the Tioga Theater to see a movie. There were only fourteen people at the matinee. My walker almost got away from me as I didn't put the brake on after I got in my seat which gave both of us a mirthful moment.

After such a fun night, I had a terrible night and awful morning. The pain was like when I was first diagnosed with cancer. I couldn't keep my eyes open but had to use lounge chair to be able to be comfortable to rest. Then I couldn't get out of the chair without help. I had to wake Bill up to help me and he was so out of it he didn't understand my problem. I cried a lot due to being depressed and in pain, and I'm sure the withdrawal from the steroids was a factor too.

The roads were really bad but I had an appointment for my chemo and Zometa hook-up. Dr. Sheth wanted me to see heart and gastro doctors as well. I didn't think they would find anything wrong but I said I'd go. Phone calls came in today from friends as they do most days. Dan was coming to see me via a frequent flier airline ticket. I cried because I so desperately wanted to see him; he hadn't been home since my cancer diagnosis. I met with Dr. Cooke for referrals but he was blunt about my chances of survival, which he felt to be a toss-up. He was a lot less positive than either Dr. Sheth or Dr. Grethlein.

I had terrible pain when I got up due to not taking any painkillers in the middle of night. My stomach gurgled, my food tasted terrible, I felt tired and I had no appetite. Terry and Dan called to wish me Happy Valentine's Day. Craig sent me a joke valentine. Craig also called to say how much Abbey loved her Disney valentine clothes from Grandma and Grandpa for Valentine's Day. The dress-up outfits for baby Olivia that matched Abbey's were a special big hit.

Bill and I saw "Chicago" at the movie theater and had lunch at Friendly's, but I didn't have much appetite so I only ate a small amount. Both the theater and restaurant were sparsely filled with people, which was good for me. I napped from 4 to 7 PM and then just relaxed. I felt very, very cold and my skin was terribly dry.

The next morning, we had twelve inches of snow so I cancelled my heart doctor appointment. I only ached in my hips but I had diarrhea.

The next day I went to get my PIC line washed and blood taken. I was given a shot of Procrit which in four to five weeks would boost my energy level and red blood counts. Dr. Sheth said I had to have a neurological or CAT scan to check on headaches and sinus, so I contacted my primary physician, Dr. Cooke, who made the appointment.

Still feeling despondent from my talk with Dr. Cooke, I made a list of my jewelry, where I purchased it, and whether it was real or costume, so there would be a record for my family whenever they inherit it. I experienced IBS and diarrhea and had a tummy ache in the evening, so I took GasX and drank Gatorade. I couldn't sleep because Bill was snoring, so I watched *America at War* with Charles Stanley and took notes to pass the information to others via the computer. Protestors were rallying online as well as in the news, and I believed God wanted me to do my part to input some sanity into the fray. Having a life or death disease that I was battling gave me a perspective many others didn't have. I decided to battle this cancer with all my resolve. I realized that God is my ultimate means of support.

The following day, I saw Dr. Cooke, who set up the x-rays and scans for next Tuesday. He also started me on antibiotics for sinus infection. I purchased Depends for Mom, and Bill delivered them to the boarding house and sat with Mom for a while.

I went back for tests on Wednesday. Bill and I had lunch and did some shopping. We got home about 4 PM and I was so tired I slept from 5 to 7 PM. My antibiotic was giving me insomnia at night, which just meant I was exhausted during the day.

After breakfast on Sunday, I listened to Charles Stanley preach on fear and the war. I thought it was wonderful and my views exactly, all backed up by scripture. Next, I switched to the Catholic Mass while I waited for Bill to bring me home communion.

On Tuesday, the day I was to have my x-rays and CAT scan, I woke up with chills, feeling very sickly. I e-mailed Dr. Grethlein. I called Dr. Cooke but he was out of town so Mary Benz, NP prescribed Avelox instead of Biaxin. Then Bill drove me to my appointment for my scan and x-rays, even though I felt sick to my stomach and still had chills and diarrhea. The doctor said to use suppositories due to my hemorrhoids bleeding. I had my pump cleaned and got a shot of Procrit.

I had my heart tested the next day. My chest hurt and my stomach was still dodgy. I followed the BRAT diet -- banana, rice, applesauce and toast -- for diarrhea. I called Dr. Sheth and he prescribed another medicine to take along with the sinus medicine.

The day after my heart test I felt good, had a good night's sleep and a good breakfast. I called Terry and told her I was doing pretty well. I found out that Terry went in proxy for me to a Healing Mass in Duluth, Georgia on Sunday and was anointed for me. Craig's pastor told his parishioners to pray for a sick person with extra prayers and Craig was doing so for me.

On the last day of February, I got up at 4 AM due to acid reflux and took a Protonix. I read for a while and then dusted. The steroids gave me energy so I did dishes and laundry as well as sorted our junk papers in the bedroom. Bill cried, hugged me and told me I was "his best friend," I never thought I'd hear something like that from him. Some good things were coming from the cancer scare; my husband was turning over a new leaf, and my children were at church and praying.

The Coburn Free librarian called and asked if I'd like some books to read. They are keeping me well supplied. One of the perks of living in a small town is that people help each other, and I have been a member of the library since I was in second grade.

On Sunday morning I listened to Charles Stanley preach on a Christian's duty during a war. I called to get "America at War" prayer cards to hand out to friends. I told the young man who took my order that I had cancer. He said he would pray for me and added that I was an inspiration. My eyes couldn't open all the way due to bloating and fluid. Mucous was draining and I'd started coughing and sneezing. Somehow I'd apparently been exposed to germs.

Dan Mieczkowski came to visit me. We cried together when he told me he loved me as his second mom. He said he'd felt his mom's and my prayers all his life, and that just sitting with me touched him because he saw Christ in me and it gave him peace.

The next day I was so weak, tired, chilled and I coughed so much that I was glad not to take any steroids that day. Dr. Cooke called to say that my brain and sinus scan were okay. The lower spine pain could have been arthritis. Myeloma was still showing in my scalp. He said to use Tylenol for the chest and hip arthritis. Later that day, I found two whiskers on my face! No hair on my head but some on my face. Go figure!

I was up all night due to muscle cramps in my legs and I couldn't move. Bill rubbed my legs and finally I was able to sit in a chair, waiting to get ready for oncology work at Lourdes.

I had blood work, Zometa, Procrit infusions and injections. I was so happy I could walk; I wasn't sure I'd be able to after last night. Dr. Sheth said I could eat peeled fruit like bananas if someone else peeled them.

Dr. Fluegel, a chiropractor, hugged me and told me he was so sorry about my illness. He worked on my back and gave me a moisture heat pad to use on my lower spine.

Dan called and wanted to know what I meant when I said I was having a bad day. (He would be arriving from Las Vegas in two days and I think he wanted to be prepared for whatever he might find.) I told him I was in pain, very weak, unable to do anything and that just sitting was uncomfortable. Nonetheless, I could hardly wait to see him.

I saw Dr. Cooke and he told me I had some myeloma in the sinus bone area but my brain was okay and so were my sinuses. I was wheezing so he put me on an antibiotic and ordered a chest x-ray which showed no pneumonia or bronchitis.

It was eight degrees when Dan arrived from Las Vegas. I was at Lourdes getting a chemo pack hook-up to take home for 96 hours of chemo. Craig, Julie and girls arrived at the house as well. I held baby Olivia for the first time and I grinned from ear to ear to see my newest grandchild. Her big sister, Abbey, was shy but took to her uncle Dan after he read to her and gave her some gifts.

The next day, Dan and I went to Dr. Fluegel as we both had appointments for chiropractic treatment. A nurse at the doctor's office told me of a tailbone pillow and I ordered two, one for use at the house and one for the car. That evening I felt "yucky" and cried. Dan and Craig took turns hugging me and consoling me. Bill kept coming in to the bed to say he loved me.

Each morning I took Protonix for acid stomach and ate an hour later as per instructions. I listened to Rev. Charles Stanley preach a sermon entitled "God Is in Control –My Assurance." I listed the scriptures and took notes. Three statements that spoke to me were that God works in every circumstance for good, nothing can touch us apart from the permissive will of God, and because God is sovereign, we can have confidence in the future. My family went to St. Francis Church for Mass and then to the American Legion for breakfast while I followed the Mass on TV and ate at home. David Franz

There But For the Grace of God

called and asked me to e-mail my shopping list for English items to him so I did. Our sons showed their parents some more computer skills, and I made my first eBay purchase. It had been great having our sons and Craig's family here. Craig and Julie asked Dan to be Olivia's godfather at her baptism in July.

I slept lying down again. I thought, God Bless Mike Fowler and the prayers for sleep that he said for me.

The next day, Craig's family left to go home to Malone, New York. Bill was exhausted from cooking and cleaning. Dan waited on me as I was worn out.

Dr. Michaels's bill was still screwed up. Bill and I had words over the bill because Bill didn't want to call the insurance company so we argued in front of Dan, which was awful. I cried. I think Bill was so tired he wanted to ignore the bill. Bill took Dan to the airport. No supper for me as my bowels and gut were bothering me. I woke at 2:30 am and had yogurt, fruit and two popsicles.

I didn't have much appetite and now weighed 156 pounds, down from 162 at my first weigh-in at the hospital. Krys called and was coming to visit us from April 5 to 12 so we could celebrate my birthday. I did some laundry; that was a big deal for me to be up and busy so long. My sinuses were bothering me, and I kept wheezing and wetting my pants -- how lovely.

Bill and I got up early so he went to Sam's Diner for breakfast. I think it is so wonderfully "small town" that patrons have a key to the diner, put on the coffee pot and visit before Sam, the owner, arrives. Sarah called to check on me and Sandy and Jim stopped by with an inspirational tape and some lemon drops. The sugar free lemon drops helped my dry mouth so much. Joanne Murphy sent soup and chili from the Parkview Restaurant. Walt Beardslee stopped by with a box of chocolates. These are examples of "small town" relationships which gave me such comfort.

I saw Dr. Sheth who said my blood work was good but I needed to take steroids for two more sessions. It was possible that on March 25 I would be admitted to Lourdes Hospital for chemo.

Bill and I got medicine and other items for Mom, after which I took a nap until 5:30. Then Rachel helped me walk on the street from our house to the corner and back home again. I was exhausted and it was only five houses and lawns to and fro.

The McFadden family had Masses said for me in Knock, Ireland and at Our Lady of Snows, Illinois. On a trip to Ireland, Bill and I had visited Knock, where the Virgin Mary had appeared. The church had crutches, wheelchairs and walkers abandoned there by people who experienced physical healing.

On St. Patrick's Day, I baked cookies, did laundry, sat on the porch in the sun and read the paper, after which Rachel walked me to the corner and back home again. I decorated the house for Easter. My legs were so weak it was hard to walk upstairs to where my decorations were stored, but I wanted to see the house decorated for Spring before my transplant in May.

Laura Tormey, MS, R.N. N.P from Upstate Medical Hospital in Syracuse sent me a schedule in the mail as well as information on what I could expect when I was there. One of the things she sent was a booklet on reducing the risk of infection. Bill and I washed all the bedding and curtains and vacuumed everywhere as well as dusted as per the booklet from transplant unit that says dust in the house is bad for my recovery due to spores.

Kathy's brother-in-law came down with multiple myeloma the same week I did. He never got well enough to get his adult stem cell transplant as he came down with pneumonia and passed away. Infections are very dangerous to cancer patients who have an impaired immunity system.

I couldn't sleep again that night, and got up at 5:30. Whenever I awoke in the night, I felt a strong call to pray. That night, I felt called to pray for my country, the military and our allies, and for the liberation of Iraq and against terrorism in United States of America. I still had a sore butt and bleeding, so at a decent hour I made an appointment with Mary Benz, my nurse practitioner, for Thursday and called Sandy Ross to pray for me.

Sandy said the mission at church had been praying me up all week.

Chapter 8: Spring Brightens my Life

On the first day of spring, my sister Sue took the cruise that Krys and Terrence, Bill and I were supposed take until I got cancer. This made me feel sad that we couldn't be there. My spirits were lifted when Diane came to my house and trimmed my hair and my wig for me.

The following day from 1 to 3 AM, I experienced diarrhea, pain and bleeding. I took a Vicodin for pain relief. When I passed stools I panted just like in childbirth which helped with the pain. I called my family doctor and he referred me to Dr. Steven Hassig.

Dr. Hassig checked me over and found a large hemorrhoid and wanted to do a colonoscopy on me within a week.

Later that afternoon it was 69 degrees. In March that is really warm for New York so I wanted to step outside. I stepped, all right. I fell down the garage steps at my home. I hit my head and got a large goose egg, skimmed my shoulders, broke my collarbone, and hurt my pelvis, where I had broken a bone last August. I hollered for Bill, but he was too far away in the back yard to hear me. Avon, who lived next door, heard me and she ran over to help me up and ran out back to get Bill. I iced everywhere I could. I saw Mary Benz, NP, who checked me out from my fall. I was okay except for the damaged parts I mentioned above -- plus I had broken blood vessels in my groin and buttocks from falling on cement steps. The temperature went back to a normal of 39 degrees. Go figure.

The following morning, banged up as I was, I got up at 5:30 AM for my trip to Lourdes to prep for my colonoscopy. I drank medicinal solution from 7 AM until 11 AM and then napped. I certainly got my bowels emptied out by running to the toilet from drinking all that awful tasting stuff. I had the procedure done at noon. The doctor removed a polyp. Internal and external hemorrhoids were found. One large outside hemorrhoid had a blood clot that was removed by Dr. Michael Barrett who fit me into his schedule at once. We told him we knew his family and he did everything he could to be helpful. He told me to use a washcloth to wipe my anus, take antibiotics and use gauze packings. I rested at home and ate some soup. Bill was worn out from waiting around all day, and my mind was confused quite a bit. It was very humid again and my collarbone was swollen and painful.

As I had been hurting so much, I decided to find tapes of joyful times. Toward the end of March I went through all my tapes and found a tape from 1984 of Dan playing the trumpet to "Onward Christian Soldiers" and Christmas carols, which was a Christmas gift from Craig. I played another tape of Dan, age twelve, announcing 1989 Little League games with Jim Raftis, the commentator, and a tape my sister Sue had made on which she prayed the rosary. The tapes gave me such joy and took my mind off my health. I played Christian music and said all of the decades of the rosary with Sue's tape so it was like we sisters were praying together.

Bill went shopping for two items at a grocery store and called me three times to help him find the items. I made myself a turkey Reuben sandwich but dropped it on the floor. Bill got mad and I got upset. I fed myself most of the time but was not always very steady with my hands and feet.

Around the beginning of April I saw Dr. Barrett, who found a fissure (a cut in the anus). This was what bled when a bowel movement stretched it. I was given a nitroglycerin/petroleum jelly combination to put around the fissure. Dr. Barrett said, "You will get a headache from the medicine." I thought that was weird; medicine for the anus makes your head ache?

After we left the doctor's office, we picked up my Aussie mate, Krys Rowell, from the airport. We had mounds of snow and only she was thrilled. Krys had lost her voice and was wearing a mask in case she was coming down with something that would affect me. I explained how important it was that I avoid germs and viruses, as my body couldn't fight infection. Both Krys and Bill reassured me they would be very cautious. They wiped down doorknobs with Lysol and stayed away from close contact with me.

A few days later, Dr. Barrett called as he was concerned about my getting an infection if I had the chemo while the fissure was not healed. Dr. Barrett suggested surgery. Bill, Krys and I left home at 7:45 AM for Lourdes Hospital. I had blood work and my PIC line cleaned. Then I saw Dr. Barrett who said the fissure was no better so he scheduled me for surgery on April 10. I went back to the Oncology Department and had my IV of Zometa and Procrit, each costing about $1700+ before insurance.

I couldn't eat after 8 PM on April 9 due to my surgery the following day. It was scheduled for 3 pm but we had to be there by 1 pm. My surgery was finally done at 5 pm and after going to the drugstore we got home at 8:45 PM. I had a very painful anus packed with gauze. My throat was irritated due to the tubes placed there because of the surgery. I was on Cipro for infection and Darvocet for pain. My shoulder and collarbones hurt and there was swelling near the collarbone and up my neck. Bill complained he was beat due to the long day of sitting and waiting. I'm the one that endured surgery and he was "beat." I think women are stronger in this respect.

Bill had a sore throat and kept using my bathroom which annoyed me due to the fact that he could give me an infection. I locked the bedroom door so he had to go upstairs to the other bathroom.

The day after the surgery my butt was hurting and I was taking pain killers. I used a Sitz bath three times a day as well as stool softeners. Pat Franz stopped in with bakery bread, rice pudding and a small roasted turkey. Bill was not feeling well, and complained about the house and the "stuff" (clutter) in it. This certainly did nothing for either of us except cause stress. After forty-some years and three children, we were bound to accumulate "stuff."

Lynne Mieczkowski, a neighborhood friend, stopped in to give me a blanket she made for me to take to Syracuse because I said frequently I was cold.

April 14 was my 61st birthday. I received lots of cards. Sarah, Sally, Krys and I had Rueben sandwiches that I made and shared a cake that Bill had purchased. We visited and I showed the girls the tape of Olivia that Craig had sent. Tyler and Molly called to say, "Happy Birthday," as did Dan, Craig, Abbey and Terry. Bob Franz stopped by with a card. At times I had wondered if I would make it to this birthday, and here it was.

My tooth was aching and I didn't know why, but thought it might be from the birthday cake icing. Later that day, Dr. Schachter, our dentist, found an abscessed tooth and recommended a root canal. He was going on vacation so he sent me to a dental surgeon in Cortland which is sixty miles from home. The dental surgeon worked on me and gave me a reduced charge for the service due to my cancer.

We got home about 7 PM after going to the drugstore for antibiotics. Dr. Cooke's office had left a message on our answering machine. I <u>needed</u> to call him back tomorrow. Around 10 PM my painkillers stopped working so I took some Tylenol. The next day my face still hurt where the root canal was done.

In the morning I called Dr. Cooke's office. Dr. Cooke said my collarbone on the right side had lesions in it which probably weakened it and hence the fractures in the clavicle near the joint by the sternum.

Sarah and Dan both called to check on me. They cheered me up as I had felt so depressed and I'd been crying. I wondered if it was because of my medicines.

Four days later I had an appointment with Dr. Barrett who said my rectal surgery was healing nicely. Bill checked with Dr. Sheth, who said I could use ibuprofen for the inflammation and pain of the root canal. Bill and I drove to Cortland, New York again and saw another dental surgeon. This dentist told me the pain should go away in a couple of days. The next day my tooth and jaw still ached. I called the Cortland office and still another dentist wanted me to come in. I was weak and it was so tiring traveling sixty miles to and fro so many days. However, the pain was really bothering me, so we went and he cut the gum to relieve pressure. He also put me back on Vicodin after a consultation with Dr. Sheth. I still had some pain but not as bad as before, as blood and pus came out of the incision. I had to rinse every hour with salt water.

I had blood on a wipe from my rectum so I called Dr. Barrett's office. They said to call on Monday if the bleeding continued, so I waited the weekend out to see how it progressed. It's pretty bad when you hurt from your head to your butt and all areas in-between. Give me a break!

Flowers were delivered so I had Bill take them back to the florist as I was still not allowed to have real flowers. Originally, I'd asked the delivery man to take them back with him, but Bill hollered at me and said he'd do it. Then I remembered something a relative said about accepting husbands where they are and praising the Lord in the situation.

On April 20, Easter Sunday, Bill went to Mass and then brought communion to me. I tried to sleep but the phone kept ringing. I knocked my jaw with my hand attempting to answer the phone and it hurt so much that I cried and cried. Bill picked up a turkey dinner, apple pie and shrimp from my sister-in-law, Pat. We had a wonderful supper. Craig called to tell me Abbey prayed for "Grandma Franz, Great Grandma Hulbert and for the magical world of Disney" which gave me a good laugh. I could always use some laughs.

I went to Lourdes and had blood taken. I waited for four hours to find out that I was being admitted to Lourdes Hospital where I was given a chemo treatment. They woke me up to give me a sleeping pill, and after that I got lots of great rest even though I was awakened all night for tests. The next day I had no appetite and ate a small lunch and lots of pills. I couldn't use my left hand to write due to the tubes so I wrote in my journal right-handed. Afterward, I could just about read it! Bill helped me cut up my dinner meat. I ate a little mashed potato and two spoonfuls of apple crisp. I listened to EWTN and said the Chaplet of Divine Mercy. The next day, I was still having trouble with constipation, chills and lack of appetite but I was discharged even though the paperwork took about two hours until I could leave for home. I felt crappy and hurt everywhere.

Another day and I had another shot of Neupogen. These shots stimulated my cells to multiply so that when I went in for the blood storing process there would be lots of cells available.

Even though it was Sunday I was back at Lourdes for another shot. As usual I received several phone calls from family and friends.

I saw Dr. Sheth for follow-up and admitted to Lourdes from April 20

There But For the Grace of God

through May 7, 2003. I was having chemo to get prepared for my stem cell transplant, but since I had developed fever and infection, I was in hospital longer than normal, which is usually only four days. Pat and Dick Franz must have been scared by my appearance and feared I'd go into a coma or not last through the night. They talked to my sister, Sue, who called Craig, who called us, afraid we were keeping information from him. Bill reassured him that I was doing fine even though I didn't look like it. When Bill's cousins, Joe and Sally, visited me the next day, Sally had tears in her eyes the whole time. I must have been in a bad way as far as my appearance.

When Bill brought me home, he was so eager for me to see our new roof that had been put on the house while I was in the hospital. I asked him why the roofers put on a different color than what we ordered. Neither Bill nor the roofers had noticed the discrepancy! The supplier ordered the wrong stuff, but told us that if we would accept the new roof as is, we would be offered a discount and new shutters. We accepted.

Bill went grocery shopping and bought chunky applesauce so we put it in the blender. He says there are so many products and so many differences that shopping is not a good time for him. He had a carry-out order of burgers and chili for lunch but after one whiff of it, I ran to the bathroom and threw up. I've noticed that with chemo I can't handle perfumes or scents of any kind.

The following day, Bill and I were off to Syracuse at 6:30 AM for an 8:30 appointment. My lungs, heart and blood were tested. Then I talked to Dr. Sara and to NP Laura and we drove home.

Bill was exhausted and napped three times. He was so spaced out. My illness seemed to be getting to him. He needed to lighten up so as not to get sick himself.

The next day we were off to Syracuse x-ray to get a Neostar Catheter put in my chest. This was the first time I have ever been under a tent for surgery. It was not too painful except for the numbing shots. Rebecca, my nurse, was so kind and informed me she was famous for her margaritas. I wondered when I'd have a margarita again. The Neupogen shots made my head feel like a wind tunnel and someone was tossing balls back and forth. When I returned home, I called Rachel over to the house to get me some Tylenol from the kitchen as I was too light-headed to get out of bed, and Bill was outdoors mowing the lawn.

Again, I received another Neupogen shot at Lourdes – a quick trip. When we got home, Sarah Hall stopped over, but she'd only been there a few minutes when a visiting nurse, Carol, came by to show Bill and me how to clean the catheter. I felt crappy and laid down a lot that day. That evening, Sarah stood in proxy for me at St. Patrick's healing service. God bless her for thinking of that.

Carol J. Franz

On Mother's Day, all of my grandchildren talked to me. Craig and Daniel called but as Terry was here visiting me, she and Bill took cards and candy over to my Mom. Molly, my Southern granddaughter, told me she had written a report on stem cell research for school. I hoped she stressed the wonders of adult stem cell human successes.

The next day, Terry drove me to Lourdes Hospital where I got my last Neupogen shot and Nurse Sandy removed my PIC line. Nurses Barb, Sandy, Lisa and Laura hugged me and said to let them know how I did at Upstate Medical. Terry did the laundry and helped me pack my hospital bag. Sarah and George paid a donation to have St. Patrick's Church youth group put flamingoes in our front yard. Terry and I each wore my turbans, stood by the flamingoes and had Bill take our photo.

Bill and I were up at 4:30 AM and ready to leave at 5:30 for Upstate Medical in Syracuse. I had received growth factor shots called Neupogen for two weeks which increased the number of stem cells in my blood. Neupogren can, if needed, make adult stem cells leave the bone marrow space and enter the blood. As I had bone marrow cancer, they took from my blood. The process of separating the stem cells from the blood also involves two arm veins; one for the blood to enter the machine for separating out the adult stem cells, and the second to return the cells not needed back to the patient. From 7:45 until 2:45, I was hooked up to a machine that circulated my blood every 45 minutes until a number of cells were collected. I napped on and off and had my own private nurse, Wendy, who by the way, loved margaritas also. As Bill and I were driving back to Owego, Wendy called us on our cell phone to say they needed 5,000 micro liters per bag of adult stem cells and they got 33,000 so they have plenty of adult stem cells and I won't have to go back as planned to extract more cells. They will freeze and store the extra cells in case I ever need them. We got home to find that someone picked up the flamingoes from the front lawn.

I heard from Laura Tormey, NP that my transplant admission would be Friday, May 16, 2003 and my adult stem cell transplant set for May 20.

Chapter 9: Darkest Moment in the Valley of the Shadow of Death

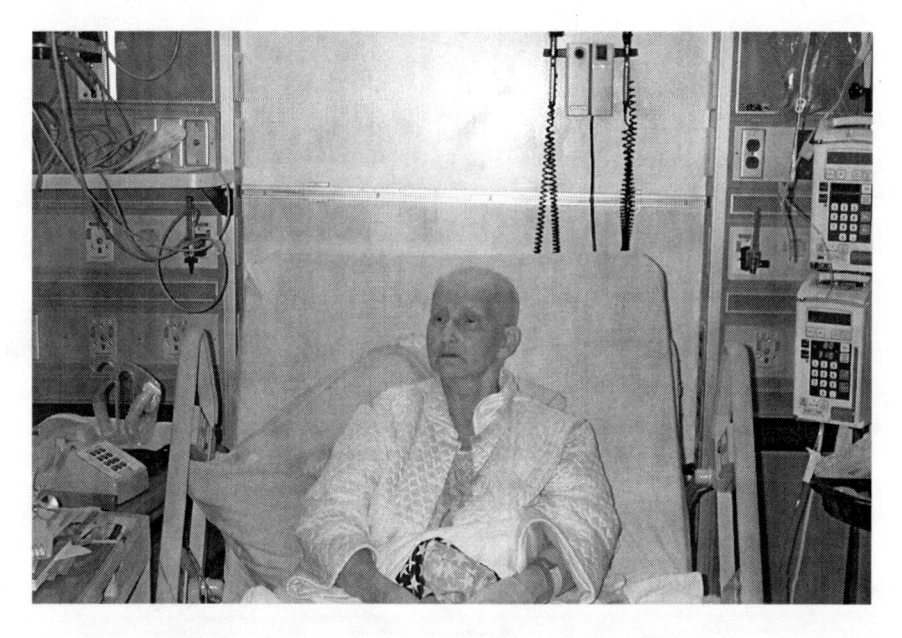

Between May 16 and June 4, 2003, I was hospitalized for twenty days for my adult stem cell transplant procedure.

My first day in the hospital, I was given a massive dose of chemo that lasted fifteen minutes. This was to destroy any remaining cancer cells. I lay in my sterile room for five days for the chemo to leave my body. I felt as though I was in the "valley of the shadow of death" since I was so weak. Five days later, a syringe containing my adult stem cells was inserted into the catheter in my chest, slowly releasing them over a fifteen-minute time span. Thus I was physically reborn on May 20, 2003. The adult stem cells traveled to the core of my bones, set themselves up, and began slowly growing a new immune system and blood supply in me. My nurses called me a miracle!

The pages printed here are my own hand writing and show the course the treatment had on me from day 1 to day 20, as well as other things that happened during those days.

Entered Upstate

5201 - order additional snack

Cafe: 2nd floor

FRI May 16
Had chest x-ray & EKG

get weighed while in bed. Have my own shower.

464-2778
consults after discharge

Friday May 16 - 4

4-4947 to order free video

Called Mary Lou & left phone #
  Kathy

Called Craig & talked & gave him # abbey wanted to talk to. Olivia coughed.

Apartment empty — 2 bedroom we can use instead of B&B

Mary Lou called. John(88)'s sister 69 yrs old died of cancer.

May 16 pm   had a strawb chfe
cup of ice cream

Have been sneezing & coughing late evening.

May 17 Day-3 Sat.

Massive Chemo .... talked to Bill & Mary Lou & Al brought me groceries from Wegman's. Mary took my laundry home to wash & will bring it back later in week.

Tried Walking after breakfast 20 laps. 1/3 mile (regular BM at 19 laps.)

2- 20 min naps due to nurses doing bloodwork etc. Nurses awfully loud laughing, etc so played earplugs & music & dozed off.

My newspaper order didn't go thru so my male nurse (Danny) left his & I gave him my $4 towards deliveries for my older.

Received my first mail from Betsy Meyers. Danny first child of mine to call.

Wants us to take some border trips to spa + gold resorts, roast beef dinners 2 nights $79 each.
 Alex Nimmo.
Sending me Harley Davidson dew rags.

🛁 Shower + then 4:00 Mass Sat.
F. Bebel
"God prunes his living fruit"

Rested, ate, talked on phone to Bill. He's bringing M. Lou's wood carvings up to hospital. She has invited him to stay there anytime. She is doing my laundry.

May 18 Sunday -2

Craig called. Terry called. I walked BK after. Had 3 bowel movements. After my shower I tried to move the chair and bruised my middle toe. Got the Syracuse Sunday paper.
 I called Bill at 8:40 and he was writing a check for Mass.
 Having chills. Hoffman hot dog tasted good for lunch with mustard + relish. Took maalox prior to eating. Also had small portion of tin soup + orange sherbet.

Bill called from J.C. Wegmann's. No small boxes of cranberry juice to be found.

Bill brought me cards from Donna (check "30") Joanne, Joe + Teddi + Brenda. Bill took a nap.

Mary Lou + Al visited with Bill + I. She pd me by check + Bill gave her the Cat Meow stuff.

Mary Lou called around 8:30. I told her Bill went home. He didn't know what to do even though he has an overnight bag packed.

Monday Day-1 May 19th

Called Sue at 7:30 am. She has arthritis in her feet. She's going on a diet + trying to stop smoking which will help.

Talked to Dr. wright about taking protonix. Laura checked - hospital doesn't have so Bill to bring mine in.

May T— 20   Sat 24   Wed 28
    W 21   Sun 25   Th   29
    Th 22   Mon 26   Fri 30
    Fr 23   Tues 27   Sat 31
                           Sun June 1

I called Sarah Hall and we made tentative plans for a visit on Friday 23rd & 30th.

Evelyn the cleaning lady asked me lots of questions about being a Christian. Evelyn my nurse is a preacher's kid and we talked of faith & God for about 20 min.

Al Seymour brought my laundry to me & I had a nice shower.

~~Diane~~ Fuile called this morning.

Bill came up & spent time with me. A nurse told me to eat crackers to soak up stomach acids.

Craig called 8:15pm. He plans on coming to see me next weekend.

adult Stem Cells 8 AM transplant

Tues. Day 0 May 20

Diane's cousin stopped to see me.

8 am <u>blood stem cells</u> went back into my body. They felt cold

Played my Jesus tapes.

Laptop computer marked up today ~~————————~~

Al got me signed up on computer.

sent to the desk top

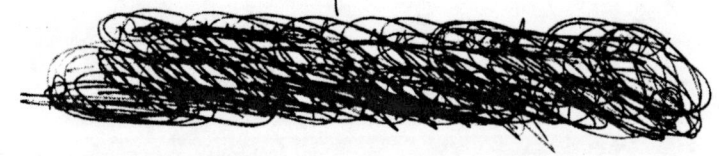

~~████████████████~~

Walked 3 times.

Fr. Bedel brought me communion.
Mary Lou & Al visited.
<u>I called Dan</u> & Brenda.

Got a neupogen shot!
Bill called again.
Got a card from Katie in hospital

Wed. Day +1 May 21

Diane called & told me of her place in FL. Sounds too desolate for Bill & me. Just fishing no beach. Near Everglades.... lots of mosquitoes & sharks.

Bill called from car.

People send greetings.

Taking pills is a hitch sometimes.

Food tray came wrong for BK but trying a hotdog for lunch.

11:45 Mass with Fr. Bedel

Called Yvonne in Bursledon. She sent me postcards of Plymouth.

M.L. called Craig & Abbey called. Terry called.

Mail from UK only took 3 days!

Thurs. Day + 2 May 22   60°

Bill stayed overnight at Mary Lou's. He got here about 10 + stayed until 2:45. We talked, napped, watched Price Is Right. He listened to his earphone music. I dropped my cassette player but he fixed it.

Mucous but I rinse. Chills. Walked some in room due to construction in outer hall way.

Had ½ a sloppy joe for lunch + ½ cup tom soup.

3pm tummy grumbling so I'll eat some crackers.

Bill took home laundry + will send it up with Sarah + Sandy on Friday. Bill is going to Hank's to get my shoes. Bill purchased about $900 worth of air conditioners for the house. After paying for them + for the shutters we'll have about $500 left over.

He wrote checks + paid some bills.

Nathan the 18 yr. old next door cried he didn't want to be "here" + pulled some of his tubes out. ML + I prayed for him. He is crying now at 7:20 pm. Kathy, a Catholic Chaplain stopped to talk to M & I. She asked about mulitple myloma & high protein as her doctor said she had a 50/50 chance of having it. I told her to go see Dr. Gentile at the R.O.C. for a second opinion. She may just be pre cancer as her blood readings flucuate & her bone marrow was good. M & I received communion.

At 7:20 I prayed in tongues towards Nathan & all became quiet in his room.

I left Diane a message about no perfumes & hairspray.

I called Dan to tell him I had a good day.

Walked 19 min but got tired. Danced in bed to praise music.

~~Kathy~~ called & is coming up on Sat.

Fri May 23 + 3 Day   rainy

Felt shitty. Holly woke me at 3:30 due to having trouble drawing blood. Chills, gut ached but

~~Silvio James~~ Eastwood, ~~$~~ > Wegmann's Ate yougert for BK.

Felt awful but took pain bill + listened to Christian music.

Sandy Ross, Sarah Hall, + Diane Fierle ~~stopped~~. Prayed with me. Diane gave me new pj's. Girls went to lunch + I went to sleep. I was still asleep when Diane came back but awake when Sandy + Sarah came. They prayed over me and we all prayed for Nathan.

I threw up my spaghetti supper. I read the paper + listened to Spiritual singers.

Kathy, the Chaplain stopped but because of throwing up did not receive Jesus.

~~Sat May~~ 4 May 24

Plathlettes done.

Kathy & Bill called from Wegmann's

Pat Franz ~~called~~

Kathy brought me a Maxine stuffed toy but it isn't new so couldn't ~~keep it~~. Nat' still doing well. We prayed for him.

I showered, napped, had tom soup for supper.

Craig stopped & brought me a video and photos of the kids.

I slept on ~~off~~ until 10:30 pm

Watching Jody Foster ~~~~ in the ling. I.

not good day

Mem. Day Wkend

Sunday May 25 Day + 4

Need blood, platelets + red. (white)

dozed on + off all day yesterday

~~Sarah & Neal called~~ I cried.

~~[scribbled out]~~

Pain was OK   Kathy + Bill came.

Very sick from transfusions, + pained

Doing   Tried to get friends to order

I got cards.

Mike + LeeAnn stopped.

Mary Lou took
Craig
dozed all night.

Mem. Day

Mon. May 30th ~~Say the~~

Had platelets & red blood transfusions. Being my pain ~~medicine~~ in IV and lots of my medicines ~~Dana were in~~ ~~the~~ ~~medicine~~ with the

Craig held my ~~ha~~ ~~kiss~~ hand during treatment.

Tell Bill ~~Mom is grumpy~~

Talking to myself ~~goo~~

~~Hedric~~ I'm heavy drugged and can't ~~write~~.

Talked to MaryLou

Tuesday May 27　Day +7

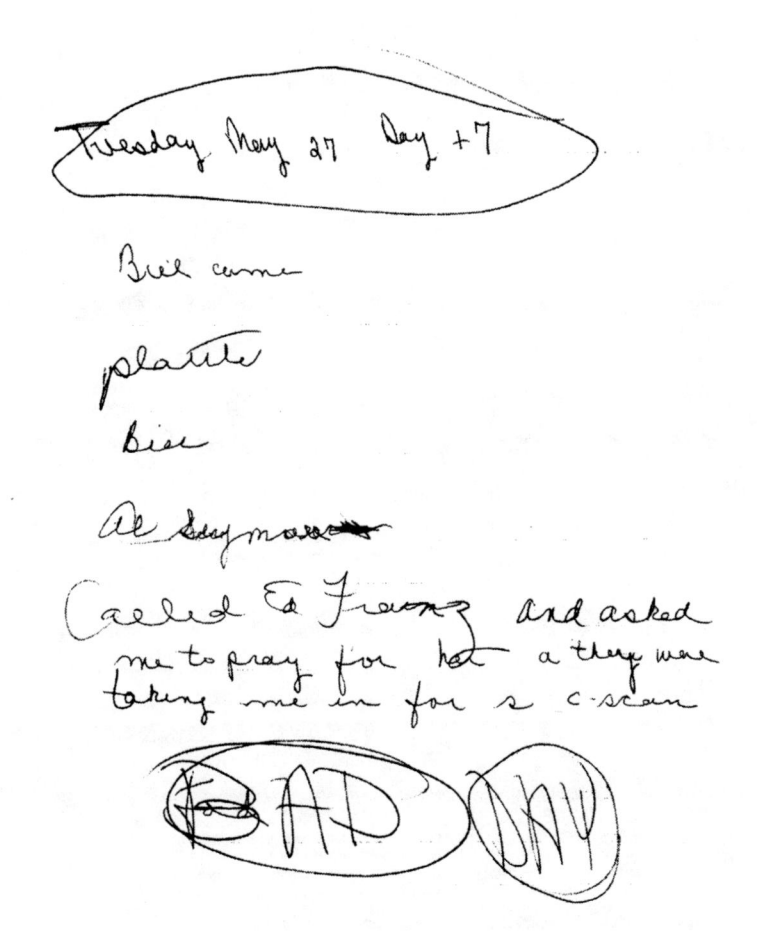

Bill came

platlets

Bili

Al Seymour

Called Ed Frank and asked
me to pray for her as they were
taking me in for a c-scan

BAD DAY

(Bled Day +8 May 28)

WB Cells at 0.2 (200 more)
R. 22.8   getting a transfusion

Bill called and ~~to the~~
talked to Dr. J. Wright.

Sarah visited

Marlenée ringing.

~~Kathy~~   101 fever

Can't print or ~~write~~ to ~~bed leg hurts~~   Bath

Bill & I walked.

ML ~~ou~~ I visited for 2 hrs I slept most of then

BAD DAY

Thurs + Day 9 May 29

one equals 1,000

WBC 1.2
HCT red 29.3
Platelets 22

Had chest tube cleaned. All the doctors say I look great but I'm tired

I did my walk + also

Peeing again from Lasix drug because I don't think enough

Eyelene told me my blood configurates have to at ANC 500 before I can go home.

Line out
1104

Mary Lou stopped in. Craig called + cried because I was doing so well. Perry called + we discussed her telling her the kids need to see me. He was pissy but called back & said okay he could take them out of state.

Tyler wants to come to Omega for four weeks. He'll have to pitch in and help

Terry made have found a 3rd story 2 bedroom apartment out in the country a little but rents is $700. Her insurance for therapy has run out but she goes to some group session I offered $60 when she needs it.

Kathy called & woke me up at 8:00.

Nurse took my temp of 101 something.

Weight 155 4pm

Threw up in night chunk of mucous that had broken away. I felt good after that. Nurse Sue stayed with me the whole time.

Friday, May 30 +10

WBC 3.5
HC 28.4
platletts 15

Sarah Hall called & is coming up.

Bill called & is coming. I feel so tired

Walked, bathed. Getting platletts

Bill, Sarah & George were here.
Heidi gave us the "sex" talk among others for going home.

Kathy Backman called from AZ. She'll visit around June 24-26

Called Dan, Craig & Mom.

Saturday May 31 Day +11

WBC 6.1
Red 24.9
Platelets 23

Diane called. Bill called. Terry called. Received 3 cards.

Unhooked me from all IV tubes at 1:00.

Bowels are similar to all cancer patients due to chemo.

Kathy & Bill came to visit. Dan called about Valco & his job hunting & sharing an apartment. Dan made me laugh. He is so precious to me.

Fr. Bebel brought me communion at 6pm & gave me a green scapula & book.

8:30 fever of 101.7. More blood work to find cause. Dr. Wright will evaluate as it could be just my white count & red blood cell spots on skin.
Heidi found a rash on my back.

60

~~Monday~~ Sunday June 1 +12

WBC 9.1   5-10 normal

Hct 31.2

plt 13

fever 101

Sandy Ross + Sarah Hall surprised me 2:30 with a visit.

Mary Lou came about 4.

Craig, Danny + Maggie Iseminger called. Pat Franz called 6:30pm.

Tom soup for supper

Mon., June 2 + 13

WBC   3.6
N+   32.4
Plt   31

Bill called + I started throwing up my yogurt breakfast. Dr. Coyle talked to Bill and me.

Craig called + woke me again.

Nurse Sue visited with me. After I walk I'm having a milkshake.

ML called tonight. She said she talked to me this morning but I don't remember.

June 3 Tues. Day +14

   WBC   2.9

   HCT   34

   PLT   31

Sarah called twice to see what dr. said.

Bill called.

Dr. Coyle + Laura said I can go home tomorrow.

I get weepy + my breathing is different.

Bill came.

Diane + Kathy called.

Terry + the kids called. I cried + asked the kids to come see me.

Engl/Seam. March 1998

June 4, Wed. Day +15

W   2.8
Hct   34.4
plt   31

Is Zumeta a form of chemo? No

20 days in hospital
Going home today!

June 9
W   3.1
Hct   37
Plat   45

June 16
W   3.2
Hct   33
Plat   30

June 23
W.   4.39
HCT   29.9
Pletlets 33.4

June 30
W.   3.99
HCT   31.1
PLT   50.1

Chapter 10: Hope and Healing

The day after I came home, I returned to Syracuse to see Dr. Sara and have blood work done, which showed an improvement. Bill and I had lunch at Friendly's of soup and a shake as swallowing was still not all that easy for me. When I got home I returned all the calls that the answering machine had picked up. Each call was from someone new; it surprised me that so many different people were concerned about me. The post was filled with cards every day and the e-mails grew as well. God was so good to me and showed me how good people are as well.

Rachel walked me down the street the next day. I was a little wobbly as I was still pretty weak. I thanked her for bothering with an older person and she said she owed me plenty. Didn't I remember the times she missed the school bus and I'd drive her to school, or the times her rabbits got out and we searched for them or the clothes I gave her or the snow days when I'd take her and her sisters in until their parents got home from work? I guess I just took doing stuff for other people for granted as a way of life, and didn't dwell on it.

Bill took me out, just for a small ride and not to a doctor's office. That used to be considered a "small thing" but now everything is special to me. Then we walked to visit our neighbor which consisted of the length of four neighbors' properties. It seemed a long walk for me but is really very short.

I had been home from Upstate Medical one week before I went to Sam's Club with Bill to walk inside a large building due to the rain outside. I received a phone call from my British prayer group, who were so pleased to hear I was up and walking around!

Sunday, Rachel again walked outdoors with me. Bill brought me communion from church and as it was Father's Day all the kids called to talk to Bill and I spoke to them as well.

We went to Syracuse again the next day. My white count was up but the other blood counts were down so the Neostar catheter had to stay in my body. Dr. Sara didn't seem worried but I was disappointed. My lunch consisted of a milkshake at an A&W Drive-In. I was tired when I got home so I slept for about half an hour. I had an Ensure for supper. Whoopee!

I received a touching, prayerful letter from Art Reynolds which made me cry. Art worked for the Village of Owego, New York when Bill was the Mayor of Owego. The letter was filled with prayer and scriptures of healing. (See letters of encouragement) I read it over and over again.

I went to the grocery store with Bill. I talked with people who told me Bill needed a lot of help in the grocery store when I was so ill and that they all tried to help him. Mother's caregiver called to say Mom was getting worse, so Bill stopped over to check on her. I still couldn't go there due to my low immune system since I couldn't take a chance of contacting a virus or infection from any of the elderly people there.

The next day, I went with Bill to get our swimming pool water tested at Johnson's. We stopped at a restaurant and bought soup. I got a burning pain in my throat and esophagus and went outside as the pain was so incredible that Bill said I turned white in color. Connie Schumacher stayed with me until Bill brought the car around. As soon as I got home I took an antacid and got some relief. I felt depressed but looking at Dan's photo cheered me up. I also played classical music which helped. My bones and muscles ached, but Bill said that his did too. It must have been the humidity and dampness of our weather, which I thought stunk.

Kathy came to our home with Italian bread and we all ate the lasagna and salad that Ed and Carmen Zonio brought to our home. This was my first salad since Christmas 2002 when I was told not to eat any fresh vegetables, so I savored every bite.

The next morning, Sandy Ross walked me on the street but we had to quit as people started mowing their lawns and spores were in the air. I walked on Prospect Street for ten minutes. How the mighty have fallen. I used to walk four miles a day.

Dan mailed us a letter he received from the Nevada Board of Engineers stating he passed his Engineer's Intern exam. Bill and I were so happy and thanked the Lord. After dinner of more Zonio's lasagna, Bill and I rode downtown and stopped to listen to music in the gazebo at the courthouse square and then drove around for a while to just relax and savor life. Bill and I also walked across the new bridge. I sat for a moment in one of the scenic areas where there are benches. It was wonderful to be outdoors in beautiful weather and chat with people we met on the bridge.

I don't mean to imply that I felt completely back to normal. Actually, I ached all over and I mean everywhere. I had no energy. Sarah stopped by to get my mind off my aches and pains. I read my journal to her of our time together when she visited us in England. Bill took me walking in a grocery store after he got home from a lunch date.

Sue called from Florida to say she will visit me in July. I watched Mass on TV and then Bill brought me communion from St. Patrick's. At home I ordered a Medic Alert bracelet per Syracuse's instructions. It must be engraved with "Stem cell transplant. Use irradiated leukopoor blood products only."

Mother's friend, Thelma Catlin Gale, called me from Apopka, Florida to see how I was doing. I told her the latest on Mom. Thelma said, "Hilda said you were mean to her but I understood because I nursed my mother who had Alzheimer's as well." I promised that when I got better, I would go to Florida to see Thelma. She told me she loved me and prayed for me.

The next morning, we went to Syracuse for blood work again. I had thrush so I was given another pill to take. I ate an egg salad sandwich in the hospital cafeteria. The doctors were happy that I had gained two pounds but I wasn't happy about it. I had hoped to be thinner from all this. I napped and then rinsed my mouth with water and white vinegar due to the thrush. I also took medicine for it as well.

I was up at 7 AM to say Chaplet of Divine Mercy and a rosary for Sarah, Terry and Dan. Bill and I went to the jewelry store and made arrangements to get a clock repaired; while we were there, Patti prayed over Bill and me. When Patti prayed, she shook. The Lord showed her how I will get up in the morning and do stuff like I used to. She said I would give testimony before large crowds of how God healed me, and tell my story. She also said I might write a book. I have had people say to me that God must love me a lot to bring me through the struggle to the other side and that he must have great plans for me.

I still ache but the humidity is at 86% today. I cut my fingernails but I don't dare cut my toenails until the doctor says it is okay. They don't want me to bleed due to my low platelet count. I had my first shower today since June 6. The bandage covering of plastic came off but the bandage didn't get too wet. I had my eyes examined by Dr. Williams in Owego. He said the eyes are the same as before my illness and the chemo was very good to me as it had not damaged my sight.

I attended St. James Charismatic Mass in Waverly, New York, a half hour car ride from Owego, where Papa Watts and others prayed over me for deliverance from bone marrow cancer. One lady at Mass said I have always been such an inspiration to her and others talked of my great faith. I didn't think my faith was special; it was just my faith.

I attended Bette McCormick's funeral at St. Patrick's Church, Owego. Mike hugged me and told me to never give up. I sat away from the crowd but wanted to be there as Mike and I had been friends since our high school days. Bette and he had sent me many cards when I was so ill even though she was going through cancer as well. Many people told me that I looked really good and they felt so relieved. I had a turban on as I still had no hair.

Off I went to Syracuse, New York as my red and platelet blood counts were up so I could have the catheter taken out. I had to sit up for five hours so I sat in my chair reading and dozing. I was so glad to not have the catheter any more as I was concerned about infection. Shortly thereafter, Sue Ballard drove me to my appointment with Dr. Carol Miller and to UHS for blood work. We had lunch and Sue told me how her faith had grown due to me.

We got flamingoes again! What a great fundraising idea for our church youth group and how encouraging to know people are thinking of me.

Soon after my lunch with Sue, I decided I was ready to drive myself. I only went around the block, but even that short trip made my muscles and sinuses ache. I love the people in Owego but the weather is just too painful. After I got home, I rested for a while, and then Bill and I sat at the Courthouse Square and listened to bands play. Several people came over to talk to us. The Mayor, Barb Fink, performed a wedding on the bandstand as we watched. Bill and I had dinner at Mario's and they stayed open just for us as it was after hours.

Soon it was time to go to Syracuse again, and I was officially discharged to Lourdes Hospital. My platelets are up but other counts slightly down. Dr. Sara and NP Laura hugged me good-by and said I was doing well and to go and live my life!

I was sick in the night with a yeast infection, stomach ache and diarrhea. The medicine isn't agreeing with me so I called Dr. Cooke's office and they said to come right in. I did, and received medicine that helped.

Darlene, Mom's caregiver called. Mom fell on floor and when Darlene tried to lift her, Mom cried out. The Owego Emergency Squad took mother to Lourdes Hospital. When Mom passed by the other ladies sitting in their chairs she asked, "Is this a whore house with all these women sitting around?" She cracked up the workers there. Bill and I spent four hours at the hospital waiting for answers concerning Mom. Mom is very with it at times and times she is "out to lunch."

I ached and felt tired but called my sister to tell her Mom's partial hip replacement was postponed due to fluid on Mom's lungs and her lack of oxygen. I was so tired that I had to lie down several times. We visited Mom for three hours and she was rational a lot of the time. The sharp pain seemed to have cut through the cloudiness of her mind. She asked me why I had a wig on and when I told her I had been ill with cancer, she wanted to know why no one had told her.

Mom's hip replacement surgery was accomplished a day or so later, after the fluid was removed from her lungs. I talked to Sue before and after the surgery. We were at the hospital from 3 to 8 o'clock and came home while she was in recovery. By then I was exhausted.

When I returned to Lourdes I found out she had a room for rehab at

There But For the Grace of God

Willow Point Nursing Home in Vestal, New York which was only a twenty minute ride from Owego. The medi-van took her and I followed. I fed her in the hospital and then we waited. Mom was not too clear. She said to me, "Who the hell are you?" One day, Bill and I stopped in to see Mom and watch her therapy. She actually knew who I was and did very well. Because she had Alzheimer's, Mom had no fear and no worries about being "too old" to succeed. She had therapy twice a day and eventually used the steps in the stairwell to walk from one floor to another. I was so proud of her.

I saw Dr. Sheth who was surprised to see me, especially when I told him that Syracuse didn't want me back in three months and that I wasn't on thalidomide pills. According to the International Myeloma Foundation newsletter, VAD (my chemo) wasn't being used like it had been. Thalidomide was tooted as the new, best treatment. The magazine also said you could have a second adult stem cell transplant. Not that I expected to need one–all my blood counts were up.

I had mammogram, pelvis ultrasound and bone density tests done. I went to see Mom and brought burgers and fries for us to eat in the lunchroom. An aide said she wished she was brave enough to wear her hair as short as mine. I told her, "You don't want to go through what I did to get this hair style." Several people mentioned to me how they admired me for going without a wig. I didn't even think about it. Cancer has a way of doing away with concern for your appearance. I just wanted to live.

I got Bill a new watchband at the jeweler's and Skip and Patti prayed with me. As soon as Patti took my hand, she again started shaking and praying. Skip prayed out loud for my healing. He told me how his faith had grown from mine; it inspired him. Patti then prayed in tongues and said the Lord showed her a vision of me on a stage speaking before masses of people and that I should buy a hand-held tape recorder to record what the Lord would reveal to me. I just looked at her in amazement as this had never entered my mind.

I put a thank you ad in the Owego *Pennysaver*. "Dear family and friends, Thank you for all the prayers and support given to Bill and me as I went through treatments for multiple myeloma, a cancer of the bone marrow. In May, I received an adult stem cell transplant from 'me to me' and my blood counts are steadily improving.

"There were many times when I could feel your prayer power and the touch of Jesus, Our Lord and Savior. I stand on the healing scriptures, Isaiah 53:5 and 1Peter 2:24 and claim them for my healing. I still need your help and prayers. The cause of this disease is unknown and there is no known cure. There is however, hope.

"More research is needed to find a cure and develop better treatments for the multiple myeloma disease. If you desire, please make a donation in Celebration of Carol Franz to:
International Myeloma Foundation
12650 Riverside Dr., Suite 206
North Hollywood, California 91607-3421
Thank you and God bless you, Carol Hulbert Franz"

In August I drove three hours to Alexandria Bay, New York with Kathy to spend an overnight with our friends, Margaret and Roy. This was my first big venture on my own without Bill since the transplant. We went for a ride on their boat and toured Boldt's Castle on an island in the St. Lawrence River, Thousand Islands, New York.

When we got home again, Bill and I were invited to our grand-niece Bridget's birthday party, but as she just had her immunization shots for the coming school year we couldn't attend. I had to stay away from any recently-immunized child for at least six weeks.

Our dear friend Yvonne arrived from Bursledon, England for a visit. I took Yvonne to the River Rose Café for an American version of an English Tea. According to Yvonne, "It was very nicely done." She mowed the lawn when we got home with a petrol mower as she only had an electric one in England. She loved the autumn colored leaves in our Owego area. Yvonne stayed for ten days and left for England after Bill showed her some of the sites of New York State.

I was still having abdominal and bowel-related issues, so I made an appointment to see Dr. Cooke. He who said my pain was diverticulosis and put me on Bactrim until I saw Dr. Sheth, my local oncologist again. I was to rest until the bowel got better.

Bill and I had decided to fly out and visit Dan in Las Vegas for our 43rd wedding anniversary on November 26. We hoped to stay through Christmas, and we checked out Las Vegas oncologists "just in case." When I was so ill, I became determined to visit family and friends more often once I regained my health.

I walked every day it was not raining and visited Mom three or four times a week before Bill and I flew to Las Vegas to spend the holidays with Dan. George and Sarah Hall, who were visiting their son, picked us up and we rode to Bryce National Park and to Zion National Park, Utah. The sights were wonderful as was the company. I do not take anything or anyone for granted any more.

Bill and I celebrated our 43rd wedding anniversary at the Bellagio. Our room overlooked the water show which was spectacular. We spent

There But For the Grace of God

Thanksgiving at Dan's in Las Vegas. Terry and Tyler flew in and surprised us. It was great to have some of my children together for the holiday.

Sadly, Dr. Shay called me in Las Vegas to let me know that cancer cells had been found in Mom's lungs but treatment would be too hard on her, so they were going to keep her comfortable and pain-free. But the Willow Point Nursing Home was under quarantine due to the flu. With my impaired immune system, I would have not been able to visit my mother even if I was at home. So we decided to stay where we were.

In early December, we flew to Loveland, Colorado from Las Vegas to visit Brenda and Jack Morse and spent three days catching up on our lives. She was such an emotional support to me during my illness.

We spent Christmas with Dan, his friends Vasco and Victor in Las Vegas. Dan's dog, McBain, got most of the Christmas gifts. I wrapped McBain's gifts in tissue paper so he could rip them open. His favorite was the Hillary Clinton chewable squeak doll.

Then one morning I was awakened by a phone call from the nursing home saying Mom had passed away. Hospice had been with her and she had no pain and just drifted off when death overcame her. I was so sad to think I had not been there, but I had called everyday to check on her. Thank God for hospice. Bill and I tried to get airline tickets home but nothing was available until January 6 due to all the holiday fliers. The arrangements had been dealt with years ago with the funeral home and they took care of everything. A small private memorial service was arranged for our return.

Once home in Owego, my head and shoulders hurt so badly that I tossed and cried most of the night because I was concerned it might be a recurrence of the cancer and I didn't want to be sick again.

I made an appointment to see Dr Sheth, who immediately ordered blood work. I bled like a stuck pig after my blood work so I had to soak the shirt I had on. My shoulders ached, my neck ached and I had a fever. Dr. Sheth said I was doing fine cancer-wise but recommended that I see a doctor for arthritis. On top of that, I had a sinus infection and a fever of 103. I woke up in the night with hives. When was this all going to get better?

I rested until Mom's viewing at the funeral parlor. It was just Craig, my cousin Edie, Bill and me, as Mom didn't want calling hours or a service. Mother looked so young and beautiful and at peace that even though I was sad, I could not wish her back due to her Alzheimer's.

But I was still in real pain. So next I had a physical with Dr. Cooke. My shoulder x-rays show fractures in each shoulder that were healing. Dr. Sheth and the radiologist read x-rays together and said there might have been a slight improvement but otherwise the holes, tumors, etc. showing up in bones are old. I cried a lot that day and wanted my mother.

Next I saw Dr. Michaels. He wasn't sure what was wrong with me so he scheduled x-rays of both elbows and an MRI of both shoulders. My shoulders ached when I lifted my arms.

Dr. Michaels said my x-rays, according to the radiologist, showed multiple myeloma. Dr. Sheth's office called to say that he wanted to see my x-rays and me on Thursday. I suspected that these were old lesions and the cold, damp weather was what was affecting me, but as I am not a doctor I didn't really know. I called Sarah and she prayed with me. Bill was fearful and cried. Dr. Sheth said the x-rays didn't show anything to him and my blood was good. He wanted me to see Dr. Fallon, a radiation oncologist. I saw Dr. Fallon the next day, who diagnosed tendonitis and arthritis. I was to use Tylenol, moist heat and massage. I was so happy to hear that, I called my sister and she booked us on a seven-day cruise in February in Florida.

Dr. Sheth said when I had cancer I had 1200 protein cells and after the adult stem cell transplant I had 10. The bad cells were not multiplying. Praise God.

Chapter 11: Winter Escape

Bill and I headed out on the road to Florida via Duluth, Georgia where we visited Terry and her children. I ached so much that at each rest stop Bill massaged my shoulders.

Once we left Terry's we were on the road to Clearwater, Florida where we had a hotel room booked. When we arrived we met Jim and Brenda Kelly from the United Kingdom. On the phone several weeks before, Brenda had previously mentioned a doctor on the Isle of Man who was a thirteen-year multiple myeloma survivor. I needed to hear a good survivor story and that boosted my morale. The weather was in the 70's, sunny and warm and I did not ache at all. We sat on the beach and could see dolphins swimming in the water.

After Clearwater Beach, Florida, we went to Disney World and stayed at one of the Disney Resorts. I cried on the Thunder Mountain ride as it rocked me too much and I was sore afterwards. We relaxed swimming and eating at lots of different restaurants. We spent time with Pat and Dick Franz at their campground site but mostly we hung out at the pool. Then we stayed with my sister Sue and her husband Joe in Ft. Pierce, Florida before we went on our cruise. It was so good to see my sister and to play cards, chat and relax in a warm, sunny, pleasant place.

Our Holland American Cruise took us to the eastern Caribbean. At our table, we met Bob and Nancy Campis who were from the Catskills. We had a great time, swimming, eating wonderful meals, and enjoying the entertainment. Bill and I even won the twist contest at their Sock Hop. The DJ asked how long we had been dancing together and I told him since high school in the 1950s. When Bill and I were dancing, it was filmed on the cruise ship video tape so we bought a copy. We went sightseeing in Cozumel, Grand Cayman and Jamaica on this cruise. Bill loved the fact he could go for ice cream cones all day long.. The cruise was great fun but I was ready to be back on land again.

When we went back to my sister's, I seemed to be coming down with a sinus infection or a cold or something. I wondered if it was from the cruise ship's air conditioning. I had a fever, chills and a horrible headache. I called Dr. Cooke and he prescribed an antibiotic for me, which I picked up at a

Florida pharmacy.

Bill and I decided to start driving back north. We stopped to see friends, the Fullers, and I ended up in the emergency ward with pneumonia. We stayed with the Fullers while I was recovering and then we headed out again for New York via Duluth, Georgia so we could visit Terry and the kids again. I was aching, cold, coughing and exhausted but we finally made it home by late March.

I saw Dr. Cooke two days later. He wanted me to take more medicine for pneumonia. I became a little perkier but was still coughing.

Next I saw my oncologist. My blood counts were low and liver counts high. Dr. Sheth said we'd wait a month and then see about remedies. The x-rays showed that the pneumonia in my lungs was gone. Halleluiah!

April 14 was my 62nd birthday, Fr. Watts, Bill and I prayed over each other. We celebrated another year of life.

Some of my doctors had mentioned thalidomide to me so I questioned Laura Tormey at Syracuse about it. She said that while I was in remission there was no need for invasive thalidomide. We would use it if the disease started coming back. This relieved my mind.

On May 14, Sue, Edie, Bill and I attended my mother's burial. The ground was so frozen all winter we had to wait until then. I was aching again and I believed it was the damp weather. I tried taking up walking again, but had to stop as I was hurting so much.

Chapter 12: First Anniversary of my Adult Stem Cell Transplant

May 20. 2004 was a year since my adult stem cell transplant. It had been an experience and thanks be to God I was still alive. A few days later I attended my first local Cancer Survivor's Dinner and what hope it gave me to see all those survivors!

Next we attended the Syracuse Cancer Survivors Celebration. Bill and I were given sunglasses to wear and toy harmonicas to play along with the Blues Brothers revue. We danced wearing our glasses, and a photographer who took our picture said it would be in the Syracuse *Post Standard*. It was a great color photo of us, but it said we were from Oswego instead of Owego. Oh, well, at least we had a great time.

I was feeling really down the next day; Joe, who had encouraged me in my battle with cancer, passed away after his cancer returned. I do not take a day of my life for granted and I try to enjoy every minute of every day, but those losses really get to me.

I saw Dr. Sheth and refused thalidomide. He said to wait another month before going to the dentist as my platelets were still a little low. He also told me I could take Bextra which would help the inflammation in my bones. I talked to Susan, a woman from Pennsylvania who took thalidomide and suffered permanent nerve damage. So many patients have told me not to take it unless I had no other choice.

Tyler, our grandson, visited from Duluth, Georgia and Dan was here from Las Vegas, Nevada. Craig's family arrived and we had wonderful times together. We went shopping in nearby Ithaca, played cards and miniature golf, and had some good conversations. Ty helped out so much around the house and even joined his grandfather at the diner in the morning with the "old guys." Ty also showed his grandmother a great deal of respect and I was very proud of him.

The humidity in the northeast was awful and my bones didn't like it. Craig told me when he prayed for me, he really believed the Lord put it in his mind that I would live for a long time. That was encouraging to me, as was the fact that I was walking a little more every day.

Dr. Sheth said the x-rays showed no new lesions. The blood work showed no IgA myeloma but shows IgG increased significantly which either meant my immune system was growing back or the cancer had moved to different cells. He believed that I was okay but would test the blood again in three months' time.

I had not attended daily Mass in months but one day I had such a strong urge to go just ten minutes before Mass was scheduled to begin. We prayed for a hospitalized woman from Dallas, Texas whose in-laws were at Mass. They lived in Binghamton, New York but requested the noon Mass that was being said in Owego. As we were all leaving church after the service, I happened to be standing near the gentleman when I heard him say that his daughter-in-law was having an adult stem cell transplant that day. I told that I also had an adult stem cell transplant and I'd survived for one year and three months. I was able to answer questions for him and my appearance encouraged him that his daughter-in-law could survive and have a normal life again. I gave him my card and told him that any of the family could contact me at anytime. I know many times I was so glad I had someone to talk to who had experienced what I went through. This couple did not attend church in Owego and I seldom attended during the week. For us to be there at the same time, discussing adult stem cell transplants was God's timing. I called it a God-incidence because I don't believe in co-incidence anymore.

I was wearing a Vote Pro-Life button on my purse. The new young priest commented on how much he liked the button and I shared what had just happened between the gentleman and me. It was a sign to all of us involved that God was active in our lives. I also believed that I need to listen to that inner voice that led me to attend Mass that day.

I had another bone marrow biopsy and it really hurt. I cried this time. My thigh looked just lovely as it was bruised from my fall in our tomato patch.

John, our mail deliverer, told me how blessed he felt talking to me. He also said how happy he was to see our Bush-Cheney sign in the yard as his son just returned from Baghdad.

I love the people in Owego, New York! I just wish the climate loved me.

Chapter 13: Stepping Out

I wrote to several newspapers about adult stem cell research because the media just wasn't informing the public. People didn't seem to realize there had been so many human successes with adult stem cell research. The fact that the term stem cell got used instead of embryonic or adult confused people even more.

I attended a Church on Tap discussion at the Parkview. I shared the fact that at the same time last year I was on my death bed but thanks to the Grace of God and adult stem cell research I stood before them today. I said that if anyone had any questions about stem cell research I would be glad to answer their questions.

Also, I added, if the young lady who had questions about the war would see me afterwards I would show her in the Old and New Testament where it told that sometimes war is justified. I also answered a man's questions on partial-birth abortion.

Later that week, we stayed at Craig's home in Malone, New York for a few days. The colors of the autumn leaves were beautiful. We attended a fund raiser for the Holy Family Catholic School. The principal complimented Bill and me on our dancing. I told her Bill and I have been dancing together for over 42 years. I also shared the story of my adult stem cell transplant and we discussed our pro-life beliefs. Craig got tears in his eyes when he watched Bill dance with me. He said he was remembering how poorly I had walked up and down the hallway with him in the transplant unit at Upstate Medical.

I wrote to several more newspapers about adult stem cell research.

I was contacted by Channel 34 TV News who interviewed and videotaped me. They used a picture of me from Upstate Medical to show how different I looked before the adult stem cell transplant. The interview was on the 11 PM news on Thursday and repeated at 5:30 AM, 6:30 AM and 5 PM on Friday. Heather Hegedus, who interviewed me, gave me a copy of the interview to keep.

Jane Doty wrote via e-mail, "I was watching channel 34 and heard that a woman was treated with adult stem cell transplant. I just knew it was you. Praise God for allowing you to share your good news with so many people. I loved all the information you shared with me. May our Lord continue to heal and bless you. He had a special mission for you and you are on it -- TV, newspapers, and guest speaking so others will believe and accept Jesus as their Savior. You are a living miracle and thank you for being a fabric of my life."

Chele wrote, "I saw the news. I thought you were great. I am so amazed at your strength and faith. Those images of you being so sick really got to me. I hadn't seen you during that time and I'm so sorry for that. Praise God for His healing touch in your life. He certainly isn't finished with you yet and boy does He have a plan for you....you have a message to tell the world and you are doing it. Thank you for loving Him so much and sharing His love with us when we were kids....what a difference you have made in this world and in our lives. I love you."

Emy wrote, "Excellent newscast, Aunt Carol. You were very well spoken and the pictures totally supported the message. We are very proud of you."

Margaret e-mailed, "Hey, I know a celebrity. I wish I could have seen it on the TV."

Kathy Bachman e-mailed me from Arizona asking for my autograph. She always kept me humble.

On Halloween I called EWTN in Alabama as they were discussing embryonic stem cell research. I mentioned that I was in remission from multiple myeloma cancer and I had a new immune system due to my adult stem cell transplant. From that incident, I was contacted by a woman, Cindy, who is a leukemia survivor with an adult stem cell transplant.

Bill and I voted in the general elections and packed for our road trip cross-country to see Dan in Las Vegas. We drove through New York, Pennsylvania, Maryland, Virginia and stopped in Tennessee for a few days. We visited the McCones, Opryland Hotel, and the Ryman Auditorium for the Grand Old Opry Show. We next stopped in Nashville to check out the city sights and visited Mel Mullen, Bill's 91-year-old cousin. Then we went on to Graceland and Beale Street in Memphis.

Our next stop was at the home of Bill's cousins, Tom and Glenna Mullen, in Cotter, Arkansas where we visited for a couple of hours. Then we spent two nights in Branson, Missouri where we saw shows and ate great meals. We paid our respects at the Oklahoma City National Monument in Oklahoma. We listened to a lot of talk radio and saw some amazing scenery as we traveled. As we hit New Mexico a snow storm was predicted so we kept on going until we ran out of daylight. I love the countryside with all the plateaus, cliffs, and rock formations, and when we passed the Continental Divide we knew we were almost at our destination. While eating breakfast in Arizona, I talked with two women about my adult stem cell transplant.

During the whole trip, I wore a tee-shirt or a sweatshirt that said "Survivor, Adult Stem Cell Transplant." In each state I traveled through, people asked me questions and I handed out pamphlets telling my story and explaining the difference between embryonic and adult stem cell research. Dan told me how proud he was of me for my writing letters and attempting to educate the public.

Viva Las Vegas! We spent time sightseeing and going to shows and just hanging out at Dan's doing odd chores. We ate at a lot of casinos and play a few penny slot machines. I also made sure that I wore my "shirts" each day so that people would become more aware of adult stem cell treatments.

Craig's family arrived from New York. This was their first visit to Dan's in Las Vegas, and they would be there for four days. Everything went well until Abbey had a reaction to peanuts that somehow got in her whipped cream at the Suncoast buffet. She spent hours at the emergency room.

Bill and I had a champagne brunch at the Bellagio and then met up with Bachmans and Dan at the Orleans for some Thanksgiving Day togetherness. As our 44th wedding anniversary was the next day, we stayed overnight at the Bellagio and enjoyed some fun and the wonderful water fountain show.

I flew back to New York for a Zometa infusion and blood work. I received a note from Mom's former neighbor, Karen Warfle. "I read your article in the Pennysaver and caught a glimpse of you on TV. I appreciate and applaud your comments about embryonic and adult stem cell research. I wholeheartedly agree. Thank you for sharing your personal experience and knowledge in an effort to educate others. I am particularly glad that you are cancer-free."

I walked to town and talked with Judge Vince about my appearance on TV. The mail carrier who used to deliver Mom's mail hugged me and said she saw my story on TV as well.

I received an infusion of Zometa and, because I was dehydrated from the plane flight, I was given saline as well. I joined Sarah and George at Mass where Jim Mead spoke to me about Zometa. Zometa was being blamed for his mother's dead jaw tissue and tooth loss. He warned me to check it out on the internet, which I did.

Back in Las Vegas, I enjoyed the warm weather and sunshine as opposed to the cold of New York. We attended a lot of shows and ate at many different restaurants and buffets. At prayer meeting I met a woman who was going through bone marrow testing and she wanted to hear about my adult stem cell transplant.

On Christmas Day 2005, I celebrated two years since I was diagnosed and treated for cancer. Praise God, I felt fine!

Bill and I rang in the New Year when attended St. Elizabeth Ann Seton Parish Dinner Dance where I again shared my story of healing.

I took my records to Dr. Jean, an oncologist in Las Vegas, so I'd be able to receive Zometa and blood work there instead of flying back home each time.

Bill, George Hall and I drove to Death Valley National Park and saw the sights. Death Valley encompasses 3,336,000 acres and straddles the Nevada and California borders. We went from 3386 feet above sea level to 282 feet below. Bedwater Basin is the lowest point in the Western Hemisphere. Leave it to us to go to one of the driest places in the world and have it be flooded! Lake beds that were usually dry now had water in them, flowers were blooming everywhere and mud being scooped off the roads.

While in Las Vegas, we attended a performance by Little Richard and felt transported back in time, since these were the songs of my youth.

We also flew out to Hawaii for a week. I relished every day of health and blessings. At a breakfast buffet in Hawaii, a stranger named Cindy asked if she could sit with us. I shared my story of multiple myeloma and she told us her husband had it as well. The Lord kept putting people in my life that I could encourage.

My most memorable time in Hawaii was the bus tour of several military bases, the Punch Bowl and the AZ Memorial, a three-sided structure with seven openings, representing a twenty-one-gun salute. We were picked up by Matt in a WWII uniform with the music of Glenn Miller in the bus's background. Matt explained that the Japanese Embassy had passed on information to Japan for the invasion of Pearl Harbor, but there were two US airfields the Japanese didn't know of, Bellows and Harleva. The first airborne US Army pilots were Taylor (wearing tuxedo pants) and Welsh (wearing underwear). They unofficially shot down fourteen enemy planes, yet these men never received the Medal of Honor. Could it be because they were out of uniform during the invasion? Maybe it was because they were told not to be heroes? I took pictures of Uncle Herb, a WWII veteran who greeted people at the USS Arizona Memorial. A Sibley from Owego is interred there.

Buried in the Utah is a cremated 2-day-old twin. Her ashes were sent to her dad aboard the USS Utah which sank during the Pearl Harbor invasion. Her father escaped but her remains were still in his footlocker. On December 12, 2003, she was given a full Navy burial. A Navy diver replaced her remains after the service. I was told her sister visits there every year on December 7. Many servicemen elect to be reunited with their military brothers at death, and Navy divers place their ashes in the ship to rest eternally. All this was very emotional for me.

The Punchbowl was a cemetery formed in a crater. An Owego resident named McTamney was interred there, as was Ernest Taylor Pyle and Ellison Onizuda (a Challenger astronaut). I was fascinated to find out that $97,000 was donated by Ralph Edwards and $47,000 by Elvis Presley to help build the Arizona Memorial, which was dedicated on May 30, 1962.

There But For the Grace of God

These celebrities didn't publish the fact but quietly provided funding for this patriotic memorial.

When at Ft. Shafter I met the highest-ranking enlisted man who instilled such a sense of peace and security in me. For too many years I had taken so much for granted as far as our servicemen and women were concerned, and now I realized how blessed I was. I pray for all of them daily and honor the memory of those who gave their lives for their fellow men and women.

Soon we were back in Las Vegas where we enjoyed more sunshine, shows, and good food. I wish I could tell all cancer patients that there can be enjoyable life even through adversity. Kathy arrived from Owego and we showed her around Las Vegas. We drove to Palm Springs, California via the Mohave National Preserve and the scenery was delightful. The cacti were blooming as were the heather and daisies. On route to Palm Springs we had lunch in Twenty-nine Palms, California where we met a young lady who had her husband's Purple Heart clipped to her purse. We thanked her for her husband and his service.

While in Palm Springs we attended the Follies in a 1936 theater where the showgirls and guys are all over 55 years of age. We drove back to Vegas via Lake Havasu City so we could see the London Bridge, which was sold by the City of London, England, in 1962 and reconstructed in Arizona. We also visited Oatman, Arizona with its dirt streets and plank sidewalks and burros that roam the hills and streets, and we drove through the clouds atop Sitgreaves Pass. We stopped at Hoover Dam at twilight and then finished off our trip with an "In-n-Out" Burger. Life was good and I appreciated every day of my rebirth. God was blessing me with the opportunity to travel and experience so much!

I received a good report from Dr. Clark Jean that all my blood counts increased, especially my platelets.

All winter I had been attending the Charismatic Prayer Meetings at St. Elizabeth Ann Seton and at Joseph, Husband of Mary Catholic Churches. At home Prayer Meeting was only once a month and in Vegas I got to go twice a week. Praise the Lord.

We left Las Vegas and started our drive back to New York. We ate in Kingman on Route 66 at Mr. Dee's, a 50s style diner we'd seen featured on the Travel Channel. We did a tour of the Arizona State Campus with Vasco, a friend originally from Panama, and the next day we headed for Tucson, Arizona. There we contacted Rick Burt and had dinner with him and his wife Stephanie at the Mosaic Café. Rick, you'll remember, was a blessing to me and helped me understand adult stem cell transplants when I was first diagnosed. We drove to Benson, Arizona and stayed with Tom and Kathy Bachman, where we played cards and made reservations to tour

Kartchner Caverns State Park. After touring the caverns we had lunch at Big Nose Kate's Saloon in Tombstone, Arizona and drove through New Mexico to Ft. Stockton, Texas. Next we were on our way to San Antonio, where we checked out the Riverwalk and the Alamo. On our journey, we saw rabbits and roadrunners and the most magnificent scenery on earth. I wore my adult stem cell transplant survivor shirts and people stopped me everywhere we went to ask about them.

We visited Johnson City, Lyndon Baines Johnson National Park, Fredericksburg (founded in 1846 by German immigrants, and the site where Admiral Nimitz was born), and Luckenbach, Texas – population 7! These were all interesting and fun places. We spent St. Patrick's Day in New Orleans, Louisiana seeing the sights and the WWII National Museum. At the museum I purchased some bookmarks showing Fr. Waters saying Mass on a dock in England where soldiers were leaving for D-Day. Fr. Waters was Tom Doty's uncle and when I got to Owego I gave Tom one of the bookmarks. Bill saw a street magician from Owego performing in the French Quarter and stopped to chat with him. What a huge country, but what a small world!

Our cable car was very crowded so I sat in front and Bill in the back. I sat next to Amanda, a woman who had colon problems. She told me she was afraid to go to a doctor and showed me a mass under her abdomen. I told her God gave us doctors and she needed to see one. I shared many things with her, laying my hand on her shoulder and claiming healing for her. The Holy Spirit was strong between us. I told her I felt such peace and I would continue to pray for her. I asked her name and she wrote down her name, number and address on a box of perfume and insisted I take it. She told me she had passed up three cable cars before deciding to get on that one. We could see God's hand in putting us together. She talked of her fears. She said she wished there was a way to be able to talk with others who have shared such experiences. I mentioned the internet and gave her my home address and e-mail address.

When we went to our car the next morning, there was a note on it from a soldier who recognized our Tioga County, New York license plate. We met him and his family before we headed out on our way to Georgia. When we arrived in Duluth, Georgia we spent several days with Terry and her family. We had dinner with the Pullanos, whom we have not seen since they moved to Georgia from New York. I was in no hurry to get to Owego as they just had another snowstorm so we stopped in Staunton, Virginia and had dinner at the Edelweiss German Restaurant. We arrived back home Easter Sunday and were able to attend Mass.

Five days later, the media was abuzz with the sad news of the decline of Pope John Paul II. I went for a long walk in the warm April weather but by the time I got home I was in horrible pain. I went to see Dr. Cooke, who informed me I had shingles. Sometimes I couldn't help but cry as the pain was excruciating. I offered up my pain and suffering to God for Dan, Terry and the Pope.

I spent my 63rd birthday still housebound due to the shingles. The doctor told me he had never seen such a bad case. I received lots of phone calls from England, Georgia, Australia and New York as well as cards and visitors. Kathy and Bill had a birthday cake for me. Ed and Lynne, our neighbors, sent me a gorgeous bouquet of flowers.

A letter I wrote about adult stem cell research and its human success stories appeared in the *Binghamton Press*. I received a call from a woman whose daughter was afflicted with Wegner's Disease. I sent her a copy of the information I had and also an article on Dr. Richard Burt of Northwestern's School of Medicine. Rosemary was moving to Las Vegas and was a cancer survivor. I told her about the Comphrensive Cancer Center of Nevada, which she contacted. We vowed to meet when I arrived in Vegas again and I was looking forward to that.

Dr. Cooke said I was healing slower than he would like but I was getting better. I was still in a great deal of pain and the painkillers only took the edge off. Some people never get rid of the pain but I believed this too would pass from me. Then I found out I also had pink eye.

I sent out more e-mails to newspapers across New York State on adult stem cell research and I received more phone calls about my letter in the *Press*.

Each evening I read from inspirational books, and one particular reading really touched my heart, mind and soul about me being tired with the burdens of the day. It said to stay awhile and know that God abides with me and that He speaks Peace unto my soul. I am to dread nothing, fear nothing, and know that all is well as I wait before Him. I am being taught and being changed. The eye of my soul will be focused upon God and the insight gained will be calming and strengthening.

Also, I believe a "holy hour" can occur whenever we listen to others and comfort them just by listening.

Chapter 14: Second Anniversary

We are here to know God, love and serve Him. I must know Him intimately and Praise Him and celebrate the job He has for me. I just have to go find the ways to do that! How often do we serve our God? 1,440 minutes a day. What can I offer to God in a day? He wants my Love.

I wrote a paper on understanding cloning and stem cell human experimentation from information I received from California Pro-Life and sent out copies.

New York State was considering a bill that would allow cloning and embryonic research, and I attended an open meeting of Assemblyman Gary Finch where I spoke up concerning cloning, embryonic and adult stem cell pros and cons. I wrote even more pro-adult stem cell letters and sent them out to the *Community Press*, the *Pennysaver*, the *Tioga County Courier*, the *Legislative Gazette Albany*, the *Times Union*, the *Watertown Daily News*, newswatch@foxnews.com and afterhours@foxnews.com, plus O'Reilly, Libous, Bruno, Pataki, Hinchey, Clinton, Schumer, and Reid. I read the New York State brief on cloning embryos and stem cells.

This was the first time I had been able to wear slacks since my shingles outbreak. Thank God I was healing. When I saw Dr. Sheth, he said I'd just have to wait the shingles out. I received Zometa, my bone strengthener and my blood count reports. The white count was almost normal at 3.9; the red count was 30.5 which were 6 below normal, my platelets were 77 which were 65 below normal, and the hemoglobin was at 10.2 just 2 away from normal. Hooray!

I spent my May 20th adult stem cell birthday in Malone attending a dance recital and spending time with our grandchildren. Olivia had to wear her Belle gloves and heels to bed which gave me great enjoyment. I taught Abbey the Hail Mary prayer and also taught her how to play the ukulele that I bought her in Hawaii. The girls put on their hula outfits we gave them and performed for us. Abbey played "He's Got the Whole World in His Hands" on the ukulele. Bill's mom Sara, who was deceased, had played the ukulele and she would have been so pleased to see Craig's daughter play. When we attended Mass, everyone's head turned as Olivia's high heels clanked as she walked up the aisle to her seat. Not many three-year-olds wear princess heels to Mass. Oh, how joyful children are!

I happened to catch President Bush speaking against embryonic research and in favor of umbilical and adult stem cell research on TV today. Unfortunately, most people don't know the difference, or else they think there is only one type of stem cell research. Once I explain the research to them, they are amazed that the embryonic research is being pushed so much and they usually ask me why. I tell them there are many reasons but I believe the desire to make money is a big deciding factor in favor of embryonic research.

In Waverly, New York, both Bill and I witnessed at a Praise Mass. He told of being a caregiver and of my trolley car experience in New Orleans. I talked about adult stem cells and revealed that I was a two-year survivor.

When at the Mall, I saw Petie Meyers and her family. Petie told her granddaughter I was the one who taught Petie about having a personal relationship with Jesus. It's such a natural part of my life that I don't always realize who I have shared Christ with.

At the Memorial Day Ceremony held at the Courthouse Square in Owego, Bill and I talked about our travels to the World War II cemeteries in Holland, Normandy and the Ardennes Forest.

I sent out mailings to raise funds for Birthright. The Lord has lit a burning fire within me to work for physical and spiritual life for others.

I wrote to the *Las Vegas Review Journal*, *Atlanta Journal Constitution*, a few more politicians, and communicated with Kathy Gallagher of the New York State Catholic Conference. It seemed as if every day people asked me to contact different individuals or politicians or celebrities to tell them about adult stem cell research and so I did. While watching EWTN's stem cell debate, I sent two e-mails. I also received an e-mail from the Republican National Committee, telling me they were sending my adult stem cell comments to the Chairman and recommended I contact the local party as well. Kathy Gallagher asked me to e-mail again the *Albany Legislative Gazette* which I did, but they kept ignoring me. I also sent a letter to Speaker Sheldon Silver but it was a waste of a good stamp.

I heard a voice from the past called Randy. He shared how the "Godly Woman" of me helped bring him to the Lord. I was around him in the 70's, written to him when he was desperate, and opened our home to him when he was in high school. When he found himself lost in the 90's, he remembered me and others who showed him Jesus by the way we lived our lives. How many people never know what effect they have on others?

At Curves, a fitness center for women, a breast cancer survivor asked for a copy of my testimony. Others overheard her and asked for a copy as well. The next day more women asked for a copy. Gail, the owner, posted my letter on the bulletin board as well as the latest adult stem cell research results.

But then it was back to Las Vegas for three weeks, where I met my Aussie mate, Krys. I was so excited to see her and I wanted her to see me healthy. Our last time together was two years ago before my adult stem cell transplant. We stayed on the Strip and then at Dan's house.

Krys and I took a coach trip to the Hoover Dam and the Grand Canyon. We also spent time seeing how different all the casinos were and trying different restaurants. We used every mode of transportation on the strip and even went to the outlet malls via the city bus. We stayed at the Luxor and took advantage of the swimming pool to relax and cool off as June in Vegas was extremely warm.

Bill flew in for a few days and rented a car so we could drive Krys to Zion National Park in Utah. On the way there we saw many wild fires and ash was in the air. We drove her to Red Rock Canyon as well as Fremont Street and of course, more casinos. Two things Krys wanted while in the USA were a Cinnabon and a margarita which we accomplished a few times over. We both thought Mass in Las Vegas was wonderful and inspiring. "Sin City" Las Vegas has more churches per capita than any other United States city.

The last thing I did before leaving Vegas was to write to Senator John Ensign concerning adult stem cell research.

Our friend in Georgia, Dale White, called and requested information on adult stem cell treatment for heart trouble. He told me I was his "hero" for spreading the word about adult stem cell therapies. I e-mailed hairdressers in Vegas and New York, several senators, assemblymen, representatives and governors (and everyone else in my address book) about a Children's Hospital of Pittsburgh news release, "Breakthrough Study at Children's Hospital of Pittsburgh Found Adult Stem Cells Show Same Ability to Self-renew as Embryonic." I encouraged my out-of-state friends to write politicians in their states, while I wrote to politicians in New York. I received several "you go girl" notes from friends and groups concerning my letters on adult stem cell research. The politicians were swallowing "hype" instead of knowing the true facts concerning adult and embryonic stem cell research. Fertility expert Lord Winston of the United Kingdom said the potential benefit of embryonic stem cell research had probably been oversold to the public.

I heard a priest from Sweden give a sermon on TV. He said, "People are allowed to suffer as Christ did so that we too could bring help, salvation and spread the love of Christ. Leave planning to Jesus. Leave Jesus to open or close the way. Prepare yourself for all Jesus was preparing for you. Trust the Lord. Can He not judge your fitness for the task He gave you? Work gladly, knowing all needed wisdom has been provided, also all needed material to do my work."

This reminded me of a reading in which Pope John Paul II assured all sick, ailing Catholics their suffering has meaning in God's plan. "Suffering is never useless, dear sick ones. Human pain is precious because it has a mysterious link to Christ's trial on the cross and his resurrection. Offer your prayers to keep him the Head of the Church." I strongly felt that my time on earth had been extended so that I could share my faith with those I meet, as well as tell my story so others might be healed.

Sarah told me about one's "duty of the moment." When you are doing God's work, that can be your prayer time and petition as well. God's duty of the moment acts as a prayer.

While I worked out at Curves in Owego, a woman and I talked of God. I said God pulled me through my adult stem cell transplant. She followed me from machine to machine talking to me. I believed she saw Jesus in me but didn't realize it. When I was leaving she asked me to pray for her that she get her faith back. That was a humbling thought.

I read that Roy Schneider, the actor in *Jaws*, had an adult stem cell transplant for multiple myeloma at Sloane Kettering, New York City. I always get so excited when I read of autologous (self to self) adult stem cell transplants for multiple myeloma, especially when it's a celebrity and the papers print their story.

Yvonne wrote me from England to say no one in her circle of friends knew about stem cell research, adult or embryonic, until my letters reached the United Kingdom. Parliament slipped embryonic research past the people and as Lord Winston said, Parliament was fed a bill of goods about immediate cures with embryonic.

At July 31 Mass I became weak and sick and I sat through most of the Mass. Towards the end I took authority in the name of Jesus over depressing and repressing spirits. I found out later that my Uncle Roy was dying during that time and he passed away later in the night. Uncle Roy, a World War II veteran, used to tell me stories. His job was to cash out GIs from the service. One whose paperwork he exited was Mickey Rooney and another was Glenn Miller's drummer. Roy said due to a "snafu" of the army, he spent the war stateside in a "fountain pen foxhole." Everyone else in his unit went overseas. He often wondered if he and another GI had delivered the papers for the bombing of Hiroshima. As he had a car on base, these two were instructed to hand-deliver important sealed papers to the White House. The next day the bombing took place on Hiroshima.

I received information on how adult stem cells are being used to grow arteries, and sent them out to all the local papers and politicians, as well as my entire address book. I heard from the Binghamton Press that they were publishing parts of my latest letter. The *Tioga County Courier* published my complete letter. The *Courier* didn't edit out information as the *Press* did.

I received another "you go girl" note from Kathy in Albany as I crashed the Democratic and Republican fundraisers in my attempt to promote adult stem cell research. I drove to Hickories Park, Owego wearing my purple "adult stem cell transplant survivor" Cancer Relay shirt. I approached Congressman Hinchey as Andrew Cuomo ranted loudly in the background. I showed Hinchey the writing on the back of my shirt and told him I was one of over 300,000 people treated with adult stem cells. I also told him the letter I received from him was full of outdated research information and proceeded to tell him the newest information. I told him I realized he and his aides couldn't keep up on new technology that was coming so quickly, but that cloning embryos to have enough embryos for research was not necessary. It seemed to me that he let everything I said go right over his head. Gee, big surprise! Bystanders, however, wanted to know more and approached me with questions. One woman bashed President George W. Bush, but after I explained how during his presidency, funding had been given toward adult stem cell research, and explained more about cloning, embryonic, and adult stem cell research, she changed her views. Two different women asked me to e-mail them information.

I received a phone call from Ruth Trombley of Brushton, NY who read my letter in August 5 issue of *Watertown Daily News*. She was a seven-year survivor of multiple myeloma and wanted to talk to another survivor. She said she'd pray for me and my advocacy. My son Craig in Malone, NY said he was very touched that someone called him about my letter in the Watertown paper and said he was so proud of me.

I was incredibly honored when the Republican National Committee called to tell me I was awarded a lifetime membership; only 1,000 people are invited for membership each year. We had a really nice talk but I had no idea why they honored me.

Later I met up with relatives for breakfast. One of them, Joe, was confused about embryonic and adult stem cell researches. So I emailed him all my mailings and prepared a packet of them for Rose, my sister-in-law.

When Bill and I attended Senator Libous's Steak Roast Picnic, Jeanine Pirro, a candidate for NY attorney general at that time, came up and patted me on the shoulder after reading my adult stem cell transplant survivor shirt and said "I'm with you."

Later, a photographer for the *Tioga County Courier* took me over to be photographed with Libous and Pirro. Both held my hands and her people took my name on their tape recorder.

Dr. Keith Nichols and I discussed Type 1 diabetes and I gave him Dr. Denise Faustman's name. I sent him copies of the Pro-Life articles. Others stopped me and asked about my shirt and story so I gave them my card and sent them articles as well.

Saturday, while downtown, I ran into Patti Davis and she prayed over me. She shook with the Spirit while praying that "living rivers of water flowed from me, anointed my mind, throat, hands and heart." She said I would witness and travel all over and even have a secretary. She said to tape my testimony and to do it soon for a couple of years would not be soon enough. I would write a book entitled *There But For the Grace of God*. And God would save souls as well as lives through me.

The following Monday, CNN made an announcement about research from Harvard focusing on fusing skin with embryonic stem cells so that cloning may not be necessary. Arthur Caplan of the University of Pennsylvania weighed in on prevailing theories that by using human embryonic stem cells, damaged hearts, spinal cords, and the like may grow back. He noted that the Far East is ahead of us in cloning technology due to differences in values, making money the big stimulus.

As if in response to Patti Davis' words, I suddenly went from explaining adult stem cell research at Curves to speaking engagements at TOPS and at Rotary Clubs. But I still continued my one-on-one interventions. At the county fair in Harford, PA, I talked with a woman on Zometa who had breast cancer. Later, I wrote Brenda, my buddy who has MS, about a Canadian woman whose MS had been stopped following an adult stem cell transplant. At the New York State Fair, two workmen asked me about my adult stem cell shirt and we talked for ten minutes. Then we went to Turning Stone Casino where the cashier in the cahier's cage called me back as she didn't understand about my stem cell shirt so I explained. She was really mixed up on what was successful and what was not. Those impromptu talks gave me a lot of practice in public speaking – and I was going to need it!

Chapter 15: Shirts and Letters Tell the Tale

I picked up another shirt from Susquehanna Printers, along with a stack of informational sheets I'd had made up. Then I dropped off a copy of my "Miracle" letter for St. Patrick's church bulletin insert, and emailed copies to the *Tioga Courier*, the *Pennysaver* and to Pirro and Libous. My massage therapist also made copies and put them in her waiting room. Lisa Hollower from the *Morning Times* newspaper called and set up an interview for a public interest story. We talked of my cancer from the beginning through the transplant, and I gave out plenty of stem cell information.

I had leg cramps and pain in my hip joint during the middle of the night so I saw Dr. Cooke. He said the results of my blood work were excellent and just to apply ice.

Bill and I went to Rudin's Old Time Farm Days and Nichols Olde Home Days. I wore my shirt and people stopped and asked about it. I explained and passed out my card or gave copy of my letter.

I went to Van Horn Jewelers to get a watch battery and ended up with much more when Carol Korba and Patti Davis prayed over me. There were more prophetic words for me; for instance, they told me I must get a tape recording made of my story which tells how Jesus brought me through my cancer and adult stem cell transplant.

I was interviewed on September 7 by AP *Morning Times* reporter, Lisa Hollower. We met at Mary Dimock's home as Mary had arranged the interview. Lisa was putting before and after photos of me in the paper along with the article of my adult stem cell transplant.

The next day I was the guest columnist in the *Tioga Courier* with an article on adult stem cell research.

On September 14 and 15, 2005, the *Morning Times* in Sayre, Pennsylvania published the story and pictures of me. Lisa said she sent it out via the AP wire and no one picked it up. So much for the Associated Press passing on hope-filled information and articles. She agreed to be part of my "rag-tag army" and do all she could to spread the hope of adult stem cell research and therapies.

Bill and I drove to Canada with Craig's family for a few hours. We stopped at an apple farm where we picked apples. Bill and I talked to the owner and explained the differences in adult stem cell therapy vs. cloning and embryos.

While babysitting Olivia and Abigail, I mailed out letters to the North Country Catholic-Ogdensburg Diocese, the *Press-Republican* in Plattsburgh, Governor Pataki, New York Assemblyman Finch, the Albany *Legislative Gazette*, Congressman Hinchey and Senator Clinton, and to Lisa at the *Morning Times*.

Arriving back in Owego, I stopped at our local health store where they had put up the articles I had written as well as the newspaper story on the bulletin board.

Dr. Carol Miller's office said that my bone density scan showed a big improvement which I think was from the Zometa, the bone strengthener infusion I receive at oncology. I no longer had osteopenia in my spine and the bone density of my hips was almost back to normal. The ultrasound technician told me her uncle had multiple myeloma so I obtained her e-mail address and sent her information. Her uncle was doing things and eating things that I was told not to.

I found out the Owego Coburn Free Library put up a display of the *Morning Times* news article. Another good thing about living in a small town is that people care and do touching things like that.

Sept. 20, 2005 was my first presentation in Pennsylvania. When the waitress found out I was the woman in the Sayre, PA *Morning Times* article she asked if she could stand in the back of the room and listen to my presentation to the Rotary Club.

That same night I attended a praise and healing Mass. Fr. Boniface, from Nigeria, prayed over me and I heard him pray against bone marrow cancer. This new priest had never met me but the Holy Spirit told him what to pray. Fr. Boniface splashed water and salt on all of us and also anointed us with oil. He told us we were a spiritual foundation and to evangelize. He urged everyone to bring three people to the next Mass except for Jim Ross who was told to bring five. We all got a chuckle out of that. We all left filled with joy of the Lord.

Via the BBC I received great news from the International Myeloma Foundation. Blood cancer stem cell transplant patients are as healthy as their peers ten years after transplant. Hooray!

I received an encouraging note from Jane Murphy. "Dear Carol, Thank you for the informative article. It would be wonderful if you could get your message in the *New York Times* and or on one of the talk shows such as Oprah. I sent your article to my daughter who can pass it around in Atlanta, GA. You are looking wonderful."

St. Patrick's Church, Owego published my story in all their church bulletins.

We attended a breast cancer fundraiser called Traci's Hope. Traci was married to my cousin, Brian Gibson. While we were there, a woman came up to me and introduced me to her 23-year old daughter. She told me I saved her grandchild's life by taking the pregnant teenage mother to Birthright where she obtained help in telling her parents about her pregnancy. You just never know how the Lord will use you to help others.

I read an article that gave 32% survivor rate for multiple myeloma patients treated in 2003. Praise God for my recovery. I am glad I didn't know that statistic when I was ill or I might have given up the fight.

I received the following e-mail from Colleen Miner, Respect Life Director for the Diocese of Ogdensburg, New York. "I was pleased to read your article in the October 5 issue of the *North Country Catholic*. I thought your name sounded familiar. You were mentioned at the New York State Respect Life Directors meeting in Albany. Your information was added to the NYS Catholic Conference Stem Cell Power Point presentation. All in attendance were proud to have a New York State resident who was living proof of surviving due to adult stem cells. I am in the early stages of planning the 2006 Life and Family Conference. Would you be interested in participating as a guest speaker? Thank you for sharing your story."

I saw my ob-gyn, Dr. Miller, for a yearly exam. She told me how proud of me she was and that she had read all my published letters. She was very much against cloning, stating that it was unethical for a doctor to even consider destroying one life to save another. Some pharmaceutical companies and some media have distorted the truth. She recommended that I continue with what I was doing, as well as contact hospitals, nursing schools and pro-life groups to request a chance to speak. She also said I looked incredibly healthy and that no one would even guess that I was a former cancer patient.

I attended St. Patrick's Human Development meeting and told my story. I was then scheduled to speak at four local Catholic churches during Saturday and Sunday masses. Later in the month I made up some notices about stem cell research and cloning in preparation for my speaking engagements and took them to several places in my hometown. Some interesting conversations came about, as many people don't know the difference between adult stem cell research and cloning. During a charismatic praise and healing Mass I made an announcement about my presentation on adult stem cell research and human cloning and I was prayed over.

During that time I had to go to Lourdes for tests on my liver, as my creatine level was too high to get Zometa. I called Sandy Ross and we prayed for a good liver reading. It was a little high, so I was only able to get 3 mgs. I spoke with a nurse who said that only a few adult stem cell transplants had been done on oncology patients from Lourdes.

I gave my talk on October 20, and it was very well received.

"I am a miracle," I began, "and Thank you Jesus. I give Glory to God. Through the grace of God and an adult stem cell transplant, I am alive. I was diagnosed in December of 2002 with Multiple Myeloma bone marrow cancer, which destroys bone. My bones looked like someone had used me for target practice. I endured six months of chemotherapy and then some of my own body's adult stem cells were collected, frozen and stored. After chemo wiped out my disease, my adult stem cells were returned to my body. On May 20, 2003 I was physically 'born again.' Adult stem cell research has the blessing of the Catholic Church. Adult stem cells are found in bone marrow, placenta, cord blood, liver, brain, eyes, nose, skin, body fat and more. Pre-natal blood cells are embryonic. Post-natal stem cells are adult stem cells. I am one of over 300,000 people treated with adult stem cell transplants. There are zero successes using embryonic stem cells. These are critical times concerning stem cell research and human cloning. In Washington DC, the House of Representatives has passed a bill to permit using human embryos. You can not get enough embryos without cloning. New York State assembly has passed a bill to create human embryos for research. Now the senators have to vote for these bills to become law. Polls show 86% of Americans are against cloning. Adult stem cell researches' medical breakthroughs render inexcusable national and state efforts to tax us to fund stem cell research. Let adult stem cells work their successes. I should not be forced to sponsor killing human embryos especially when surplus embryos are being adopted, implanted and born alive to childless couples. No embryos had to die for me to have life."

Chapter 16: Westward Ho

In late autumn, Bill and I left Owego for our cross country trip to Nevada. While eating breakfast in Virginia, I met a young man in his early 20s who asked about my sweatshirt. I gave him a newspaper clipping and explained the difference between adult and embryonic stem cells. In Sante Fe, New Mexico we met a Michigan couple whose friend had just undergone a transplant. In the jewelry department of a store, the clerk made a copy of my newspaper article to give to her son, a doctor. She believed as I did! In Albuquerque, two Latino women working in another shop hugged me, kissed my cheek and shared their faith. I shared my pro-life views on adult stem cells. They had never heard of anything but cloning embryos. They asked me to write to their bishop and to the Albuquerque newspapers

All across the United States, I kept seeing affirmations of my faith. In Groom, Texas we saw the largest cross in the western hemisphere. It could be seen for 20 miles around. I lit candles and prayed in the Cathedral church of St. Francis of Assisi and the Loreto Chapel. This chapel was built in 1878 by a mysterious carpenter for the sisters of Loreto and had a miraculous spiral staircase, built without nails, dowels or supports. All these sights enriched me spiritually and convinced me I was on the path God meant for me.

By the end of October we were in Nevada. I worked out at Curves and showed them a copy of my *Morning Times* clipping. When I picked up my dry cleaning, Virginia, an employee there, gave me the phone number of a talk radio announcer to call about adult stem cell research. She also advised me to see Fr. Bob, pastor of St. Joseph, Husband of Mary, Roman Catholic Church. I spoke there with Henry, RCIA who also encouraged me to speak with a priest. I went to the office, called Father Bob's number and left a voice mail for him. I found out he was out of the country but the recording said he would get in touch with me.

As it was Election Day, I went to Republican Party of Nevada headquarters on Durango and shared my *Morning Times* article and witness with a secretary.

I received a call from Kathleen Miller, Diocesan Director of Nevada for Life. Fr. Bob from St. Joseph, Husband of Mary Church gave her my name and number. She invited me to the Moyer Student Union on the University of Nevada-Las Vegas campus, where there would be a presentation debate on stem cell research on November 21. I arrived early. The student attending the door asked about my shirt and what it meant. I explained and she said everything I was saying was news to her. Where I sat was predestined as a Parkinson's patient sat behind me and read my shirt. We talked, I gave him information and told him I'd e-mail him more in a few days. A woman asked me where I got my shirt as she too was an adult stem cell survivor. I informed her I had it made and she could go to any tee-shirt shop and have one made as well. A couple of women sitting next to her overheard us talking and asked questions so I gave them a sheet listing the many successful adult stem cell therapies compared to zero embryonic. More people asked questions and I told them my story as well as that of Dennis Turner, a Parkinson's patient treated with adult stem cells.

John Gearhart, Director of Research and Developmental Genetics Division, School of Medicine at John Hopkins University, was the guest speaker. Kathleen was invited to do a rebuttal but she was given just a few minutes, whereas the doctor had at least half an hour to speak. He said very little pertaining to adult stem cell research and really pushed the embryonic research done in animals. When he said that stem cells had helped no one with Parkinson's, the fellow behind me said out loud, "That's a lie" as that fellow had just heard me tell the story of Dennis Turner.

When the doctor finished, there was an open mike and I told my story of survival and hope with adult stem cell treatment. I could tell by his body language that the doctor was not happy I was there and speaking up. He left immediately after the presentation but Kathleen Miller and I stayed and answered all the questions presented to us. This was the first time Kathleen and I had met, but we worked well together. A young student who was in the Navy asked questions and I gave him informational guides as well. He just didn't understand why this information wasn't out in the public eye.

When Bill and I left the building, a professor of political science asked us if we'd been at the lecture. I spun around so he could read both sides of my shirt and said, "Oh yes." My husband and I talked with him for quite a while. He asked for papers which I gave him as he would like to bring up the subject in class as it pertained to politics. He confided in us views of his that he didn't want known on campus.

When we got back to the house I watched Fox 5 News to see if my "rant" was on. I had called in to rant about biased media and politicians such as Harry Reid in reference to adult stem cell research and therapies. Of course my "rant" wasn't on. I agreed with 62% of the local people polled who said they were not pleased with the way Senator Reid was doing his job.

After the news I e-mailed some of my friends about my experience at

UNLV. I received a lot of e-mails the next morning and I quote from some of them;

"Thank God! You are getting the message out to people. Irene."

"Praise God! You are doing great work…wow….I know a celebrity. Bachman."

"Congratulations on your words at UNLV. Kathy G."

"All praise to Our God Most High. Truth will win. Fannie."

"I wish I could have been there to hear you speak. Jane."

"How awesome! Praise God! Thank you for sharing your message not only with me but with the world including UNLV. Peace, Doug."

I e-mailed the *Review-Journal* newspaper complaining about the very one-sided write-up of the stem cell debate. It wasn't a debate but a set-up against Kathleen Miller.

Bill and I spent Thanksgiving with Dan and the Bachmans, and celebrated our 45th wedding anniversary with Curt and Jane Clear at a show at the Suncoast.

I met with Greg Farino to plan a stem cell presentation at Joseph, Husband of Mary Catholic Church. While I was there, I attended the Church's prayer meeting.

I saw Dr. Jean, my oncologist, who said my blood counts were great and that he wished all his patients were as positive as me. I received an infusion of Zometa. He told me that Zometa, the bone strengthener, was now being given once a year to rheumatoid arthritis patients. What great news that was to me.

Terry sent me a copy of a letter she had submitted to the *Today Show*. The winner of the contest got to be Godmother for Freedom of the Seas cruise ship, winning a yearly cruise for life. The letter read, "In early 2002, my seemingly healthy sixty-year-old mother began having extreme pains through her body. Her skull and bones ached so badly that she would lay with three ice packs at a time on her head. She was constantly exhausted, but continued to care for my grandmother who had Alzheimer's. After nine months of searching for answers, doctors diagnosed her with multiple myeloma. Although shaken by the news, my mother's faith in God gave her strength. She immediately started chemotherapy in preparation for adult stem cell replacement therapy. In the spring she was admitted to Upstate Medical in Syracuse, NY where she endured the excruciating task of harvesting her own core stem cells so they could multiply and be reinduced at a later time. Before this procedure, however, she went through intense chemotherapy to kill all the cancer cells that were throughout her body making her bones look like someone had used her for target practice. On May 20, 2003 doctors at Upstate Medical returned her adult stem cells to her body through a 'port' in her chest. She refers to this day as her birthday; she was physically 'born again.' She has had such a positive attitude going through this whole ordeal, and gave strength to family and friends who worried and prayed for her.

From the time of her first onset of pain until now, my mother has shown incredible courage fighting this disease that came close to taking her. Her strong faith in God and her doctor's wisdom helped her through. She educated herself on the disease and was adamant about using her own stem cells. Her determination has led her from shuffling on her feet, to walking with a walker, to walking independently, to now dancing, exercising, and taking long walks. Having lived overseas for a few years, Mom and Dad received many cards and letters from friends in England, Italy, France, and as far away as Australia when she was sick. The underlining current running through these letters was what an inspiration Mom was to many of her friends during this ordeal, and how their faith had grown from observing my Mom's accepting words and actions as she battled this disease. She is one of over 300,000 success stories using adult stem cell research, and celebrated her second 'birthday' last May.

The best part of my mother's story is how she has become such a crusader of this cause as she battled back until today. She gives hope to the newly diagnosed by calling them directly, giving her account of how this disease can be beaten. She has been published in newspapers from Montreal to Las Vegas, educating people on adult stem cell replacement and giving her personal testimony. She spends hours daily writing and e-mailing organizations, politicians, newspapers and magazines on the newest developments in this field as well as on her successful experience. She has spoken endlessly about the successes of adult stem cell research to church groups and organizations. She has allowed her story to be part of slide presentations around the country, and will lend herself to speak on the subject whenever asked. She has shirts imprinted with "Survivor, Adult Stem Cell Transplant" that she wears to state fairs, political rallies, festivals, and across the USA when she travels spreading information to many who are now aware of adult stem cell successes. Her drive on this has been tireless; her dedication steadfast and sincere; her faith ever stronger. My mother is truly an inspiration and would be the ideal godmother for Freedom of the Seas."

Darn, I didn't win. I could have informed many people about adult stem cell therapies and maybe saved someone's life.

Diane e-mailed me the following; "You have been an inspiration to many…..I love to share your story. I'm thinking way back to the beginning of this chapter in your life…I know you must have questioned many times, 'Dear Lord, why me?' when you were diagnosed with multiple myeloma. I am sure you are finding peace with why as am I…Your speaking up at UNLV brought tears to my eyes…my prayers are with you…I am so grateful to have you in my life."

The strange thing is that I have never said to the Lord, "Why me?" Why *not* me? The Lord suffered, and everyone does at some time in their lives. I became a stronger person for it and maybe more appreciative than others who have not had a "wake-up" call in their life.

Dan told me today that a friend asked him how his parents stayed married so long and did they still love each other? He was dumbfounded and said, "Of course, they love each other because they are still together." I told him that his dad and I made a covenant with each other and with God. Also "the family that prays together stays together."

While exercising at Curves, a woman said that I had such healthy, energized eyes and she liked the way I explained adult stem cell research. She wanted to attend the lecture I was giving at church. Linda, an attendant, also encouraged me for the way I talked about pro-life and adult stem cell research. Then the woman said I was saving untold lives by educating people. They fired me up and I spent the afternoon writing and e-mailing newspapers.

I read online that Don Ho, the Hawaiian entertainer, had an adult stem cell treatment for his heart. I wrote to his website asking if, when he was feeling better, he would advocate adult stem cell research. His family wrote back immediately with a positive response.

I believe that hope-filled people inspire and boost others. Hope-filled people receive their strength and grace from God. Jesus was a carrier and I felt inspired to do the same. Isaiah 40:31 tells us "they that hope in the Lord will renew their strength." When I went to God and received hope, it gave me courage to spread hope. I must remember to rely on the Holy Spirit, not myself.

The Las Vegas St. Elizabeth Ann Seton Respect Life Group invited me to attend 8 AM Mass, rosary and then breakfast at the Suncoast Casino, to meet the group and share my testimony about adult stem cell therapies and my story. As we were in the buffet area of the Suncoast, I believe others around us probably heard what I said as well. I was surprised to see how many working and retired nurses belonged to the group.

Sandy Ross sent me copies of St. Patrick's Church Owego bulletins that contained facts on adult stem cell research. St. Joseph, Husband of Mary Church put the facts in their bulletin. I told Sandy she was part of my rag-tag army of helpers.

Christmas was quietly spent at home after attending Mass. On New Year's Eve, though, we attended the Knights of Columbus Dinner Dance at St. Elizabeth Ann Seton with Jane and Curt. Who says cancer survivors don't have fun?

Chapter 17: Still Going Strong

With the new year came new opportunities to get the word out. Greg Farina, a member of St. Joseph, Husband of Mary Church in Las Vegas, helped me with arrangements when I spoke there about my adult stem cell transplant. Greg was passionate about gathering people from all over the state to promote adult stem cell research, and wanted to pull together an interdenominational effort so big the media couldn't ignore it. He had also spoken to Richard Ziser of Nevada Concerned Citizens to join in. I had planted seeds and hopefully when I moved on to Texas and New York, people in Nevada would keep things rolling.

I wrote letters to the *Malone Telegram, Press-Republic* (Pittsburgh), *New Leader* (Staunton, Virginia) and the *West Side Journal* (Albuquerque). I mailed my testimony, cover letter and information on adult stem cell research to the *Legislative Gazette* (Albany, New York), Diocese of Tucson, Diocese of Las Cruces, Archdiocese of Sante Fe and Diocese of Phoenix, Arizona. Then I sent letters and photos to *Rising Tide*, the newsletter of the National Pro-Life Alliance, and also to Good News Publishing.

I decided to pray for car drivers who sped past me to recognize that they were driving dangerously and slow down. It was better than getting upset or muttering under my breath. How little they know that they are placed at the cross of our Lord.

On Bill and Elvis's birthday, Jan. 8, I attended Justice Sunday III via satellite. Sponsored by Focus on the Family and the Family Research Council, this mega-event was held in Philadelphia at Greater Exodus Baptist Church and I watched it at a Vegas church. The event's organizers stand for religious liberties and families. We were asked to pray for our President, senators, persecutors and peace in Jerusalem. Senator Rich Santorum spoke on the constitution "of the people, by the people and for the people." I learned the Liberty Bell has Leviticus 25:10 engraved on it. Dr. James Kennedy of Coral Ridge Ministries spoke of our guarantee of a religious people. Dr. Alveda C. King of King for America, Inc. spoke as well. I heard that 55 signers of the US Constitution were men of God. David Barton told that Jefferson was a child of the King. During the first 150 years of our nation's history, religion was okay. Sixty years ago the Supreme Court took anti-religious actions. Alan

Sears told how the doctrine of "separation of church and state" was not in our Constitution. Jerry Falwell warned that secular humanists were trying to take over; as an example, the Indiana House of Representatives are no longer allowed an opening prayer using the words Jesus or God.

I e-mailed *Albany Times* reporter Odato, Senator Libous and Governor Pataki after Kathy Gallagher sent me a "heads up" that universities and foundations dealing with diseases like Parkinson's were pressuring legislators to put funding for embryonic research in the New York State budget. It had been a busy day, yet I baked Bill an applesauce cake with cinnamon icing for his birthday and also picked up Dan at the airport!

The *Binghamton Press* printed my letter, "Adult Stem Cells Save Lives." I made tapes of myself to hand out to people. I also wrote to Bill and Melinda Gates Foundation to ask for funding for adult stem cell research, especially funding for Dr. Faustman's research on Type 1 diabetes. Ann Marie, a Vegas acquaintance, had a friend who knew Jim Caviezel, the actor who portrayed Jesus in the film *The Passion of the Christ*. She wanted me to write and she would have her friend send my note on to him in the hope he would promote adult stem cell research. I never heard anything back.

At my appointment with Dr. Jean I found out that my blood counts were good, as were my liver and lungs. He prescribed medicine to help my coughing.

I loved a section of President Bush's State of Address and copied down an excerpt. "A hopeful society has institutions of science and medicine that do not cut ethical corners and that recognize the matchless value of every life. Tonight I ask you to pass legislation to prohibit the most egregious abuses of medical research, human cloning in all its forms, creating or implanting embryos for experiments creating human-animal hybrids, and buying, selling or patenting human embryos. Human life is a gift from Our Creator, and that gift should never be discarded or put up for sale." I praise God for his servant, George W. Bush!

Weather on this beautiful January 18 enticed us to ride to the Valley of Fire, the oldest Nevada state park, established in 1935. I loved the gorgeous red sandstone formations with unique names like Beehives, Clark Memorial, Fire Canyon, Seven Sisters, Elephant Rock, Petrified Log and Mouse's Tank. Mouse's was named for a renegade Indian who used the area as a hideout in the 1890s.

I was still coughing but I wasn't letting it stop me as I believed it was just sinus drainage, so I attended a Mass for Aborted Babies at Guardian Angel Cathedral of Las Vegas on January 22. Jane, her mother, Mary and I sat in the front row. Bishop Pepe blessed me after the Mass and told me he was working with the Council of Bishops against embryonic research. I told him I'd be a "show and tell" if need be. He encouraged me in my mission. Two nights later I gave a presentation at Joseph, Husband of Mary Catholic Church telling my story and promoting adult VS embryonic research. My friends Doug and George Hall were there. George still had holy oil on his hands from the earlier healing Mass so he put his hands on my head and anointed me with the oil. Kathy Miller mentioned that the Bishop was considering having me speak at the United States Conference of Bishops. When I returned to Dan's house, his dog McBain sensed I was "under the weather" and lay down next to me. He is the sweetest little ole dachshund and I love him.

Bill and I left Vegas on a road trip to Santa Barbara, California. It took us seven hours, which included stopping for a lunch at the really cool Peggy Sue's 50s Diner which is eight miles north of Barstow on the I-15 Freeway. After we checked into our motel in Santa Barbara we walked along Stern's Wharf where we heard seals barking. We roamed State Street, visited Santa Barbara Mission and drove through San Marcos Pass to Cold Spring Tavern for lunch. It used to be a stage coach stop and is heated by fireplaces so it was fairly cool as the temperature outside was only 59 degrees. We stopped at Cuchuma Casino, Solvang (a Danish community) and then back to Santa Barbara where we stopped at Trader Joe's. All this brought back happy memories of our times here in the past when Bill worked six weeks a year in the area representing IBM.

I talked to a young woman who had a stroke and then developed epilepsy. Her doctor mentioned an adult stem cell transplant for her but she was afraid. She said she'd go home and research adult stem cells after talking to me. I hope I learn someday just what she decided to do.

Bill and I took to the road on our way to San Diego. We roamed Old Town, attended Mass at Immaculate Conception Church and ate in a café called The Living Room which resembled (you guessed it) a living room!

At breakfast we met a couple from Las Vegas. They were unaware that umbilical cord blood is adult stem cell. Bill and I also met a pro-life couple from California. She took my card and said she wished I could speak to her Pro-Life Group. I said I'd travel, expenses paid for me, to talk anywhere. Five years ago, I'd never have imagined myself being in demand as a speaker, but God works in mysterious ways.

Chapter 18: Texas, Here We Come

On our last day in Las Vegas for the year, Jane called and told me our hairdresser was talking about me at the party they attended. The hairdresser told of my adult stem cell transplant and how I was contacting people. I imagine she informed many that evening that were clueless about adult stem cell therapies and research.

Dan was in the process of moving to Texas, and Bill and I left to help him. On the way we stopped off at Bachman's in Benson, Arizona. We spent the night in a John Wayne-themed bedroom after playing a card game called, "Screw Your Neighbor." Kathy informed me that the *Tioga Courier* printed one of my letters.

We got Dan, McBain and belongings settled in Round Rock, TX. Friends called from Owego to say that at St. Patrick's Church people signed a petition for adult stem cell research.

I found Curves – the same fitness center I attend back in Owego -- near Dan's new home and showed women there my photo and told the story of my transplant of adult stem cells. Sometimes my boldness even surprises me, but I was trying to save lives.

I listened to PBS, where there was an interview with Christopher Scott, author of *Stem Cell Now*. He is from Stanford University and engaged in biotech embryonic stem cell research. The PBS show *Fresh Air* was moderated by Terry Gross. Some facts were stated that I didn't believe were true. Adult stem cells were not rare as was stated. The more than 65 therapies using adult stem cell research and zero human therapies utilizing embryonic stem cell research were not mentioned. Nor did anyone tell how nasal adult stem cells have enabled some paraplegics to gain movement and experience feeling in their bodies, or how in test trials diabetics and Parkinson's patients have been helped by adult stem cell research.

I think we should use our tax dollars for adult stem cell research as that is what works. Adult stem cell transplants have been done successfully since the 1960s. Adult stem cells work as well as embryonic ones, according to a study in Pittsburgh. Found in bone marrow, blood, eyes, heart, liver, skin, and body fat, adult stem cells are the core of who we are.

Embryonic stem cells are unstable and are more prone to rejection than

Carol J. Franz

adult stem cells. Embryonic stem cells have caused teratoma tumors, seizures and viruses in human experiments. Adult stem cells have less chance of rejection and don't cause tumors or viruses.

I called the Laura Ingraham Show about stem cell research. She mentioned the Leslie Stahl *Sixty Minutes* piece, which in my opinion did a hatchet job on stem cell research by interviewing only pro-embryonic professors and doctors, who skated around the truth. I said, "I am Carol from Owego, New York, an adult stem cell transplant survivor." When I was on the line, I told of surviving multiple myeloma via a transplant at Syracuse Upstate Medical Hospital, and answered Laura's questions about it. She called me a miracle.

I quit watching *Sixty Minutes*! The show had mice that can walk due to embryonic stem cells. Why didn't they show the humans treated with adult stem cells that were walking with braces and walkers? I guess that would have affected their agenda to promote embryonic instead of adult stem cell research.

I watched C Span where US House of Representatives Congressmen Phil Gingrey, R-Georgia and Roscoe Bartlett, R-Maryland discussed stem cell research. I have met with Gingrey several times and he posted our photo on his Georgia information website. I also wrote to an Austin plastic surgeon who advocated collecting adult stem cells from liposuction body fat.

I went to Curves and met Roni who was wearing a St. Margaret Mary's Church tee-shirt so I asked about the church and its location. She asked about my shirt, too, and as I explained she called me a miracle and hugged me. Together we prayed for guidance and wisdom for me and the book I was writing. I met another woman there whose daughter had a bone marrow adult stem cell transplant for leukemia.

A new priority on my prayer list was the work on my book to give hope of God's healing grace to more people than I can reach in person. I believed we are just now figuring out how God made us with our own repair kits in our wondrous stem cell make-up. They have been within us since the human race began!

I met with an oncologist, Dr. Brian Shimkus at Lone Star Oncology, and had my blood counts checked. The doctor read my counts and suggested having an x-ray but Bill said we would do it back home. The doctor told us to be sure and get in touch with my regular oncologist as soon as possible when we got home. Hmmmm.

Donna, from St. Margaret Mary's Pro-Life Group in Cedar Park, TX, asked me to speak on March 24 from 7-8:30 PM on adult stem cell research and my transplant story.

I wore my "Survivor" shirt to Curves again and a woman asked me about it. She had a family relative who had a fetal (embryonic) stem cell transplant done in Canada for Parkinson's disease. He then developed a brain tumor. She told me how he hated President Bush and blamed the President for his health issues. Embryonic stem cells create tumors in people, yet doctors try to get people to risk their lives with experimental embryonic stem cell therapies. How sad and yet how pathetic for this patient to blame the President for his problem when it was Bush who was pushing for adult stem cell treatments that actually help people.

I received more St. Patrick's, Owego bulletin inserts from Sandy Ross and e-mailed them to two Catholic churches in Las Vegas.

Chapter 19: Election Day in Texas

I wore my purple "Survivor, Adult Stem Cell Transplant" shirt with jeans, and we drove to Crawford, TX, population 631. It was an hour and ten minute drive from Dan's. As we pulled over so I could take a picture of the welcome sign featuring President George W. Bush and Mrs. Laura Bush, there were three people there doing the same. Our fellow photographers were a woman from Fair Haven, New York and a retired military man and his wife who were now living in Texas. After our initial talk, we ended up at the same shops and had lunch at the Coffee Station. The place was full of media so I chitchatted with a group from CNN. I purchased some things at Yellow Rose of Texas on the Lone Star Parkway in Crawford. The clerk in the store told me of her sister who had a bone marrow adult stem cell transplant but didn't follow her doctor's instructions so she didn't look or act as healthy as I did. Also her sister did not think positively, which I know is so important.

Bill took my picture with cut-outs of George H., George W. and Barbara Bush. After wandering in shops we ventured down to the Crawford Fire Station to see if George and Laura were voting. Barricades were set up and we had to stand back 100 yards so we waited a couple of hours and visited with the others waiting.

There was one lone protestor and whenever he shouted out negative comments, the crowd of about 40 people all cheered for the President or sang patriotic songs. I was interviewed by Matt of WACA-TV who asked why I was there. I said, "Because I wanted to thank President Bush as his administration was the only one to ever donate funding for adult stem cell research. I am alive because of adult stem cell research. I really like him." I was thanking God, too but I didn't say it for fear they wouldn't show the piece on TV if I mentioned God.

I showed my photos of the before and after adult stem cell transplant throughout the crowd and also to some members of the media. Everyone there said they didn't know anything about adult stem cells. Sometimes I felt as though I was spitting in the ocean, as so few are aware of adult stem cell research and treatments!

We saw the helicopter fly over, and then shortly after that the motorcade made its way to the fire station. We saw the President and First Lady enter to vote. As they left the polls I saw Mrs. Laura Bush very clearly as she was by the car window nearest to me.

Bill and I drove out to Prairie Chapel Ranch but we were stopped by very nice Secret Service Agents who said we couldn't come any closer. We went back to the Coffee Station where a man from Lubbock, TX asked us what was going on in town. While Bill explained, I gave the fellow information about adult stem cell treatments.

On our way back to Round Rock we stopped in Salado, TX and ate dinner at the Stage Coach Inn. This is where Jesse James, Sam Houston, George Custer, and Sam Bass -- among others -- are reputed to have stopped. The Inn stands at the crossroads of the Chisholm Trail and Old Military Road.

I wrote to Laura Bush on March 8.

Dear Laura,
I do not mean to disrespect you by using your first name. I think of you as a friend, hence using Laura.

I am praying for you and your family. I defend President Bush's stand on adult stem cell research. I am alive due to an adult stem cell transplant and I tell people that President Bush's administration is the only one to fund adult stem cell research. I am very glad he does not pay attention to polls because those of us who neither live on the West Coast nor in the East Coast big cities, but in small towns through the country, believe in your husband and what he stands for, especially protecting us from terrorists.

I reside in a small community of 3,800 people (Owego, NY) but I am in Round Rock, TX while visiting our son, who invites his parents to spend part of the winter at his home in this lovely part of the USA.

I made my first trip to Crawford on Tuesday, Election Day, and was thrilled to be able to see you and the President from afar. I wear a shirt that has printed on the back, SURVIVOR, ADULT STEM CELL TRANSPLANT. I was able to share with the crowd and the media the difference between embryonic and adult stem cells. For example, there are over 65 human successful therapies with adult stem cells and none with embryonic. Also adult stem cells don't cause tumors as embryonic stem cells have done when used in human experimental situations.

Enclosed are copies of what I pass out to people. During the

2004 elections I had several people tell me that they changed their minds and voted for George Bush for President after I explained to them about embryonic VS adult stem cells. The media says he is against all stem cell research which is bogus.

I am writing a book, *There But For The Grace of God: Surviving Cancer with Adult Stem Cell Transplants*. When it is published I hope you will allow me to send you a copy.

One of over 300,000 adult stem cell success stories,
Carol Franz

Roni mentioned to me that when we were at daily Mass and I offered a prayer petition for "those going through a crisis of faith," she felt the Lord touch her. I do know that when we held hands during the Our Father and as I silently prayed in tongues, still holding her hand, I could feel the Holy Spirit working in her.

On Sunday, Bill, Dan and I had brunch at The Oasis and margaritas at Fins on Lake Travis. Daniel booked flights for the three of us to visit Disney World when Craig, Julie, Abbey and Olivia would be there.

On March 24 at St. Margaret Mary's Church in Cedar Park, I gave my talk to a small group of people which included Dan and Bill. Dan learned just how sick I had been. It was his first time to hear me speak on the cancer and on my transplant of adult stem cells.

Dan took Bill and me to the Commerce Street Bridge to see thousands and thousands of bats swarm out from under the bridge and ascend into the evening sky. This happens every night about dusk. We had some great Texas BBQ and packed for Bill's and my journey home.

We attended our final Mass in Cedar Park where Fr. Charles Van Winkle (no relation to Rip) was a guest missionary. After Mass I gave him copies of my handouts. When I left he shook my hand and said, "Jesus shines through the light in your eyes." I was so amazed to hear him say that.

The next morning, I cried because my head and shoulders hurt like they did when I had cancer. The humidity was 73% in Round Rock.

Chapter 20: East is East

I anointed Dan, prayed over him and Bill, and we left Round Rock, TX on our way to meet up with my sister Sue, cousin Katie, and their spouses in Tunica, Mississippi. We stayed at the Hollywood Casino but checked out all the casinos and the countryside for a couple days. When we left, we stopped by the birthplace of Elvis Presley in Tupelo, Mississippi before arriving in Duluth, GA where we stayed with Terry, Tyler and Molly. I tried Curves of Duluth and told my story there. The owner asked for articles and copied them. I built memories with the grandchildren around the card table and looked at their artwork and compositions from when they were little.

I relate all these wonderful trips in the hopes that patients suffering from cancer and other diseases treatable with adult stem cells gain hope that they too may be able to travel again and enjoy life's pleasures.

But what was this? We arrived back in Owego and it was snowing! This is why I don't love New York! I had 199 messages on my e-mail. I clicked on Disney Travel Planner and had a message that our reservations had been upgraded to a one bedroom villa in Saratoga Springs Resort and Spa. I called and accepted the upgrade. A villa usually runs $343 a night but we will pay $110 as that is all we were scheduled to pay at All Star Sports.

I also received a letter today from the Bishop of Las Vegas.

Dear Ms. Franz:

Thank you very much for your correspondence of March 14, 2006. I am forwarding your correspondence to Ryan Hall, Our Diocesan Pro-Life Coordinator.

I wish you well and assure you of my prayers as you continue to offer hope and education to those who are suffering.

Wishing you the very best, I remain,
Sincerely yours in Christ,
Most Reverend Joseph A. Pepe, D. D., J.C.D.
Bishop of Las Vegas

After praying the Chaplet of Divine Mercy, I rode my bike to morning Mass for prayers for the soul of Dorothea Baker. After Mass I talked with Steve as it had been thirteen years of survival for him since his heart transplant. Glory to God!

Another former classmate, Marie, told me she was diagnosed with leukemia. The doctors told her she had five years to live. Why do they do that? I have another friend who was told a two-year life span and she was going on five years of survival. Bill says the reason is "CTA" – to cover their ass from being sued.

I received a letter from Fr. Charles Van Winkle, Austin, Texas.

> Dear Carol,
>
> May the love, joy and peace of Jesus our Risen Savior be ours now and always! Thank you for having shared with me your two articles regarding your stem cell miracle. Both articles are very well stated -- clear, concise and convincing.
>
> How encouraging you are promoting the truth and debunking the myth. May our faith in Jesus daily continue to grow. Please pray for me.
>
> "I shall pass...through this world but once. If there is any kindness I can show or any good that I can do, let me do it now, for I shall not pass this way again."
>
> And to you, love and prayers,
> Fr. Charles, C.S.C.

Fr. Charles also enclosed a prayer card called IN THE BEST COMPANY.

"And Jesus says, 'I will not leave you orphans...The Kingdom of Heaven is within...I am with you always.'

"On your word, Jesus, at this moment I call to mind your abiding presence within me and will continue to do so, especially when I am tempted to believe I am alone. For it is true: You are with me always, at all times, as my God, my Brother, my Savior, and my very best Friend.

"It is to you I can speak, knowing you will without fail respond to me with your love and strength—your rest. And at this moment you are saying to me, 'Come to me, you who labor and are burdened, and I will give you rest.'

"Jesus, help me more fully to accept and live according to this saving and fulfilling reality of your abiding and loving presence within."

There But For the Grace of God

After praying another chaplet, a rosary, and using a moist heat pad and "tens machine" on my aching muscles and bone, I went to Broome Oncology for my blood work. I believe the more I trust in Jesus, the more I receive from him.

Don't ever say I let anything get in my way or stop me. While I was waiting to hear the results of my tests, I hopped in the car with Bill and sped north to spend Easter with Craig, Julie, Abigail and Olivia in Malone, New York. When we got to Craig's, he and Julie asked us to please come for Christmas which would be our first Christmas there since the girls were born. Bill and Craig ordered me a laptop computer from Dell as a birthday gift.

On our way back to Owego, Bill and I stopped in Brushton to meet Malcolm and Ruth Trombley. Ruth had angina plus multiple myeloma, but she was a fighter. She was over 80 years old but attended Mass and also took trips to the casino and wasn't letting her illness control her! She inspired me!

The next morning, ooh my bones, muscles, shoulders, hips and hands ached. I saw Dr. Sheth at Broome Oncology and got a Zometa infusion. Dr. Sheth said my blood levels of bad protein had shot up from 85 in October to 385 in February (while in Texas) and in April were 720. My good blood protein had lessened. I needed to undergo another bone marrow tap, blood work and x-rays of my skeleton. I couldn't help it -- I cried. Bill said to stay positive. Dr. Sheth told me there was a new chemo out now plus pills I could take, and I also had adult stem cells still frozen in the Syracuse hospital.

Wonderful -- on top of that depressing news, my allergies flared up. I went to Mass and prayed for other cancer patients and myself. The French teacher from Owego Free Academy came by to help translate a letter from my French relatives who lived near Belfort, France. How kind of him to help me out. That cheered me up some.

After all my physical testing, I felt so tired. I took a nap but it didn't seem to help. What was this all about?

I attended a prayer/cancer teaching with Fr. Boniface Ewah. He suggested that I pray Psalms 43, 51, and 61 for cancer recovery, say a rosary for 41 days, and pray noon and midnight for twenty to thirty minutes daily. He told me to claim Psalm 118:17-19 in the name of Jesus. "I shall not die, but live, and tell of the works of the Lord. The Lord has disciplined me severely, but He has not given me over to death." I considered my 2002 multiple myeloma a discipline!

Sunday, April 23 was Divine Mercy Sunday and we attended Mass at St. Patrick's Church and had breakfast at the American Legion afterwards. When I returned home I telephoned Sue and also Dan about my white count increase. I watched the Divine Mercy Celebration on EWTN. As the world worsens, we are to pray for mercy. I told Sue of cancer scriptures, rosaries and prayers I was doing. I asked her to pray in the most positive way possible for my blood counts to be good counts. I talked to Fr. Watts and he said he would lay hands on me in prayer at the Praise Mass on Friday. I read the International Myeloma Foundation News Sheet for latest information on multiple myeloma. I was being bold in the Spirit and rebuking cancer. I made tapes of my testimony and research and also tapes of my dad's reminiscences of his youth in Owego. I also worked on my diaries for my book.

Irene, a friend who lived in Las Vegas, told me to send her a petition to take as she was going to Medjugorje. My petition was that my blood and protein blood counts would be normal and also for finances, faith, employment and the schooling of my children and grandchildren.

I finished transcribing my diaries thus far into book form. April 28 was the first day of typing my book. I wanted to get it published to inform public and to encourage other patients. I was so blessed to have so many chances at life!

I received some bad news, however, about my buddy Darlene. She was in the hospital with another problem besides her cancer. I went to church and obtained a prayer blanket to take to the Charismatic Mass I planned to attend that evening. Everyone there laid hands on Darlene's prayer blanket. A scripture card came with the blanket, "Acts 19:11-12: 'Meanwhile God worked extraordinary miracles at the hand of Paul. When handkerchiefs or cloths which had touched his skin were applied to the sick, their diseases were cured and evil spirits departed from them.' This blanket was blessed by Fr. Tom Watt's Charismatic Prayer Group."

Online I read about an 18-year-old girl from Waverly, Illinois, named Jacki Rabon. Jacki injured her spine in a 2003 car accident and the following year spent $47,000 for two and a half weeks of treatment in Portugal by Dr. Lima. She had an adult stem cell transplant of cells from her nose applied to the break in her spine. Oh my gosh, how wonderful! The FDA or the Food and Drug Administration had not approved this procedure yet in the USA. You want to bet if their loved ones received spinal cord injuries, that ruling would change quickly.

Kathy Bergmann proofread some of my book and took home the introduction and dedication and letters of encouragement to proof as well. We laughed so much and she was very helpful. Laughter always makes me feel better and healthier. Bill and I watched DVDs of the house where we lived in Bursledon, England, our trip to Isle of Jersey, Christmas with all our family in UK and family trips to Paris, France and Winchester, England. I have been so blessed. Someone asked me once what more I would like to do in my life and I replied, "Travel and attend daily Mass more often." Praise God for His goodness to me!

I visited Darlene Hayes at Lourdes Hospital and gave her the prayer blanket, anointing her with holy oil and praying over her. I also sprinkled holy water around her room and on her. We shared fears, faith and positive feelings.

Bill and I took a flight to Florida to meet Craig's family and Dan at Disney World. I struggled a bit getting around Disney World, but I did it and had great fun with my family. Cancer was not controlling me! Before flying back to Owego, Bill and I visited my mom's buddy, Thelma, in St. Mary's, Florida. We had a wonderful time and she said she hoped we'd move near her.

When I returned home, I attended noon Mass at St. Patrick's, Owego. I prayed, "Speak Lord, your servant is listening." What I heard back was "All is well, all is well" and I felt an immense sense of peace.

I wore my lime green "Survivor" shirt to the Republican Committee 2006 Annual Banquet as I was the guest of Owego Town Councilman, Don Castellucci. I met several politicians from around New York State and gave them information on my experiences with adult stem cell therapies. Later that night as I watched the local TV news, I was so obvious in the background due to the brightness of the lime green shirt.

On May 17, in the middle of the night, I was scared and cried. My muscles were so cramped from my toes to my thighs that I couldn't walk. I called out for Bill to help me get into bed. As I lay there I thought of my suffering as just such a small thing compared to the sufferings of Christ. Maybe this was what the Bible meant when it says we are called to be co-heirs of his Kingdom because sufferers share in His divine nature?

I was up at 6:00 AM due to more leg cramping. I was glad I had an appointment with Dr. Sheth. When I arrived, Dr. Sheth and Nurse Sandy did a bone marrow biopsy on my hip. I was told not to move but the Novocain wore off just as he was dissecting the bone and I cried out and raised my head. He said that my bones looked strong. Sandy asked me where I was going next and I told her I planned to go to Texas to dog sit. Dr. Sheth laughed as he had never heard of dog sitters. My blood pressured was extremely low so after surgery Bill had to stay at my side in the recovery room. I was discharged about forty minutes after the procedure as I had no side effects. We stopped at Barnes and Noble where I purchased a 2006 Christians Writers Market Book which I hoped would help me in my search for a publisher for my book. We also stopped at a store for Gatorade which had electrolytes in it. Dr. Sheth thought I was dehydrated or lacking in electrolytes and the Gatorade would help. I tried Smart Water as it had less electrolytes but no sugar in it.

Kathy stopped by so that Bill could help her book a flight to Austin, June 3-11, the same time that Dan was in Panama. She didn't want me being alone in Texas in case I got sick or had those bad leg cramps again. What a wonderful, thoughtful friend and caregiver she was. After she left, I typed for several hours and called Colleen Miner of the Ogdensburg Diocese to finalize the details of my speech to be given at the Pro-Life Conference on Stem Cell Research on September 19 in Watertown and on September 20 in Plattsburgh. I would share my experiences and answer questions after Kathleen Gallagher spoke on Cloning and Stem Cell Research.

Our granddaughters' dance recital was imminent, so we drove five hours in the rain to Malone. My backside was extremely painful where I had the bone marrow tap so I lay down in the backseat of the car for three hours. It was worth it, though; the girls did a great job. Bill and I ached horribly the whole time we were in Malone, thanks in part to the damp weather, but we did celebrate my third year of life on May 20, 2007.

However, our stay in Malone was shorter than planned, not because of the weather, but due to a phone call we received from Dr. Sheth. My scripture study message that day was John 16:7, which said "We may be called in our faith to move deeper through an illness thrust upon us. The Holy Spirit may be offering new and more profound ways for an occasion of grace and a maturation of faith."

There are no coincidences. There are only God-incidences.

Chapter 21: Guess What's Back?

Back home, Bill and I met with Dr. Sheth at Broome Oncology. He told us that I had multiple myeloma in 60% of my bone marrow and my blood count was 1500. However, my bones showed no new lesions or tumors and were strong. I was to go to Lourdes Hospital Pharmacy to fill out paperwork for Thalomid which was a brand of thalidomide. I would take Thalomid for 28 days while I was dog sitting in Texas. Then I would start the steroid and Thalomid pills when I returned back to New York State. I would endure this treatment for about four months and then have another adult stem cell transplant in Syracuse.

When I returned home I called family and friends and told them the news. Ed "Mitch" was walking past my house as I told Sarah, so I told Ed as well. He went home, came back with his Bible and had me read passages from it as he prayed over me. I called St. Patrick's Church and asked that my name be added to the prayer list at Mass and the list in the bulletin.

I jokingly said to friends, "If I'm going through this again just so my children attend Mass and my husband grows in patience, there has to be a better way!" Diane called and told me I was so amazing because of my attitude. The fact that I still wanted to travel made her laugh. That's me; have cancer, will travel! Kathy stopped to see me and when I told her, her reaction was that I didn't even look sick. I asked Joan to pray for me and she replied, "I always pray for you." Krys in Australia cheered me up and had me laughing. I love that quality in her and laughter was such good medicine.

One of the nuns at Lourdes put my name on her prayer list. I called Yvonne in England as the prayer group met on Thursday and asked them to pray for me.

I went back again to Lourdes Hospital Pharmacy where I had four prescriptions filled: Protonix to prevent stomach acid, Bactrim (an antibiotic), a steroid called Decadron, and 10 mg. of Thalomid. I had to get on the phone with Celgen, the company who made Thalomid, who asked me to agree that I wouldn't get pregnant. That would have been a *real* miracle at this time in my life since I was 64 years old. Did they think I was crazy as well as ill with cancer? Since then the FDA came out with their approval to use Thalomid for cancer. Talk about timing. If I had been in a test trial, my Thalomid wouldn't

Carol J. Franz

have cost me so much.

I heard from many, many people as the word got around that I had cancer *again*. Muriel wrote from France that she would think of me often. Colleen wrote that she was so sorry and prayed God to give me the strength to face this new battle. She would keep me updated on the Ogdensburg Diocesan talks and asked if I would like to be added to a pro-life prayer chain that had members across the United States. She closed with, "Never underestimate the power of prayer. You are in mine." I witnessed at Praise Mass about my cancer returning and asked for prayer. And I got in touch with an old high school classmate, Marie, and we shared our cancer experiences. We also vowed to pray for each other.

When I called Mary Lou Seymour, she was at her place on the St. Lawrence River. She was very positive and wanted to attend my presentation in Watertown. I was to let her know when I was having the transplant as she'd be there to help me.

I called Patti Fitzpatrick in Florida and she prayed with me in English and in tongues. "Prayers are to be used as stepping stones towards Jesus and you will live and travel the world doing God's work," she told me. "You are to avoid negative people and to complete your book as the Lord will use your book to raise an army of believers."

Would you believe there are still people who think cancer is contagious? There is so little true knowledge in the world of things like cancer.

Dan called and we had a great conversation. He mentioned he was more mad than worried about my multiple myeloma returning. Craig and he were both angry that this happened. Dan received e-mails from his friends Thomas in Las Vegas, Rosie in Phoenix and Rick in Tucson who were also angry but praying. Rick wanted me to keep him informed. He was a great help the first time I was diagnosed. Dan said he had a "date" the day I told him I had cancer but he cancelled it, explaining to the girl that he was upset and would need to reschedule.

Dr. Sheth explained all my drug dos and don'ts. I was bummed after than so I bought goodies at the bakery and had an ice cream sundae. That was brilliant of me! The steroids would help me get fat; I didn't need to help them.

After my course of pills, Bill and I drove the 150 miles to Regional Oncology Center at Upstate Medical, Syracuse on May 31. When we were showed to a room, one of the nurses sat with us. As it happened Gail and Bill grew up on the same street and knew each other. She learned from us and we learned from her about adult stem cell transplants. Next I was reunited with Kathy Romano, NP, Laura Tormey, NP and met Dr. Teresa Gentile. All three hugged me, and Laura said, "Your picture has been hanging up in our break

There But For the Grace of God

room. You look great." They were all enthused that I had been in remission for almost three years. They told me they had a male patient who had two adult stem cell transplants in Arkansas and two with them. A second should give me a better advantage and longer life span. Three years of survival was better than most of their patients. Good thing I didn't know that or I might have been afraid to do all the traveling that I did.

Bill told them of my advocacy work for adult stem cell transplants and mentioned that Don Ho's family had responded to my e-mail to him within fifteen minutes of sending it. I could tell that Bill was going into panic mode; the doctor would ask me a question and Bill would answer it, usually with the wrong data. Fortunately I had carried my medical records in my wallet for the last three years. Dr. Gentile asked if I'd had the twenty immunization shots that were given at one year, 1½ years and two years after an adult stem cell transplant for multiple myeloma. I said that I had only had a flu shot as no one had mentioned anything to me about immunizations. I also didn't know that after two years remission I could have stopped wearing my medic alert bracelet. Hey, I do what the doctors tell me! They did say I would need a pneumonia shot in July.

Dr. Gentile mentioned different treatments that I could choose from.
1. I could have another stem cell transplant using one of the bags of frozen cells still at Syracuse.
2. I could take Thalomid and Decadron (a Dexamethansone steroid).
3. I could take Revlimid which was a test trial that was available through her, but due to my trip to Texas I didn't really have the time allotted. It required 21 days of pills and had some of the same side effects as Thalomid, of which Revlimid was an offshoot, but Thalomid was FDA-approved.
4. I could take a chemotherapy drug called Velcade.

After much thought, I chose Thalomid and Decadron. My only chemo IV would be prior to the transplant. A catheter would also be inserted into my chest. They would use one of the two frozen cell bags I had stored. I'd find out in six weeks if Thalomid was killing the cancer cells. If by any chance it wasn't, then I'd have IVs of chemo.

I asked lots of questions, and Bill asked the same ones over and over as he said he couldn't get his head wrapped around everything being said. At one point, he leaned over to me and told me he was hungry. I didn't want to leave until I had all the answers to my questions straight in my head.

As we drove home, Bill complained that I had asked too many questions, but said that he still couldn't grasp it. I asked if he had read any of the information we had been given and he said no, because he thought that the doctors knew best. I replied, "This is my life and I need to figure out the best treatment because I will die if I don't. What about the different things my two oncologists said? How do you discern which one to follow?" Even though I'd taken good notes, Bill remembered some of the answers differently than I did. I told him I'd e-mail Laura when we got home. He was tired and cranky and said I needed to find other people to drive me to Syracuse because this was too much for him. I told him I don't need stress and we needed to be as patient and kind to each other as we are to our friends.

Chapter 22: Cowboys and Cowgirls

Traveling without Bill this time, I took a flight out of Syracuse via Philadelphia to Austin, Texas. Several people in all three airports asked what my shirt meant so I explained about adult vs. embryonic stem cells and how adult stem cells saved my life. I took Dan to the airport on June 3, and as he flew off I picked up Kathy who flew in from New York. We shopped, watched movies, shopped, typed the book, shopped, swam, shopped, walked the dog, exercised and ate out a lot at Rudy's BBQ. I continued my medication routine and did okay. The steroids had a tendency to keep me awake in the night so I'd send e-mails. I wrote one to President Summers of Harvard because Harvard was cloning. I carbon-copied it to friends and Greg asked if he could send it on to pro-life people. I said, "Yes, we are God's army."

I took Kathy to the airport at 4:15 AM, then went back home and slept some more. I was glad I rested as Bachmans arrived and we drove to Leander and the HEB grocery store. After I picked Dan up at the airport we had a cook-out for dinner and just relaxed.

Tom and Kathy Bachman and I checked out Lake Travis, the Oasis Restaurant and flea markets. I felt weak and tired so checked blood pressure at HEB and it was fine. I napped all afternoon and decided I needed to realize I was not as young as I used to be, plus I was battling cancer. Duh!

Then off I went, flitting around again. Dan took me to the airport since I had planned to spend some time with Jane and Curt in Las Vegas. On the plane I wore a mask and took Airborne. Again I had a chance to share my testimony about adult stem cell therapies with many people as they inquired about my shirt. Phil, a medical student from Wisconsin, gave me his internet address and told me that his university was building a $3 million lab for embryonic stem cell research. He asked that I get more information to him and to keep getting information out to the public.

While in Las Vegas, Jane and I walked, checked out Siena, ate at the Red Rock Casino where I had my favorite Cappriotte sub, played at Suncoast, saw Scintas' show at the Sahara, ate at Toby Keith's I Love This Bar and Grill at Harrah's, roamed through Hooters Casino, got my haircut by Ulla, shopped at Whole Foods, attended Joseph, Husband of Mary Catholic Church, hit the Fashion Show Mall, showed her Ohio friends the Paris Casino, the Orleans

Casino, the Rampart Casino, and Red Rock Canyon. We spent my last evening in Las Vegas on the patio at the Bellagio Fontana Lounge, watching the fountain water show over drinks and a cheeseboard. While we sat there we talked about our lives and our faith.

While flying back to Austin I felt sleepy and shaky as I was off the steroids. Those steroids gave me so much energy and a huge appetite. I was up all night due to leg cramps. I tended to become dehydrated when flying on airplanes so I went back on Gatorade.

I was interviewed while in Round Rock, Texas on June 22, 2006 by Donna Williams for *The Catholic Spirit* magazine. That day I was full of energy. Bill e-mailed photos to Donna in case she needed them for the article. Then he called to say we needed to go west next winter. I hoped he would remember that when the time came!

Chapter 23: And So it Begins

"Be in a state of grace with no sin barriers so prayer answers can get through. Jesus is your brother and friend so develop a personal relationship with Him. Instead of reacting to anger with stress or impatience, calm down, for the way we forgive others is the same measure by which God will forgive us. Ask all things of God in the name of Jesus. We are all sinners and what we do to be a better person is good but what we do does not redeem us in God's eyes. Accepting Jesus as our Lord, Savior and Redeemer and having Him stand beside us before God redeems us. We will want to be a better person if we truly accept Christ once we give our lives to Jesus. He never forsakes us or moves away. We do that by our words and actions in things like pride, temper and the garbage we put in our mind. We may go to the edge of the palm of His hand but He will not let us fall off. Don't use Jesus' name as a curse word but as a key to open many doors. Whatever you ask God the Father, pray it by finishing the prayer, 'In Jesus' name I pray' or 'I ask this in Jesus' name.' Fill your mind with prayer, especially the Our Father which is the prayer Jesus taught us. If your mind has scripture in it, Satan can't mess with your mind, filling it with negative or sinful thoughts. Start by saying it in bed at night; repeat whenever you feel stressed. Stress is physically and mentally bad for the body and brings on illness. Let go of it. God can take anything that happens to us and turn it to good for those who love the Lord and follow in His ways. Your faith will free you up. You are a unique gift of God with many talents and blessings. Think on those and not on negative thoughts."[1]

In June, as I flew back to Owego, I sat next to a woman from New Mexico who asked me to explain the two types of stem cell research as it was news to her.

It was raining and humid when I returned home and my body felt wobbly and I was breathing heavily. Bill and I went grocery shopping, but he got so worried about the ice cream melting that he left me in the store while he put the ice cream in the car. I was so wobbly I couldn't walk without holding on to him. It was scary!

We went to Broome Oncology where I received Zometa while Bill got my prescription for Thalomid, Protonix and Decadron filled at Lourdes Hospital Pharmacy. Bill was gone so long that I called the pharmacy. Bill and I went back to talk to Dr. Sheth about any other treatment as my prescriptions maxed out my insurance and we had to pay $3035 for my pills. We discussed what to do and I told Bill I wanted to live and to put the $3035 on our credit card. The pharmacist at Lourdes was a sweet man who told us to contact our insurance company and if that didn't work to call a lawyer. I was crying and Bill was upset. We needed a lot of money for the treatments and stem cell prescription. Bill called the insurance company from the hospital and I called Sandy Ross to pray with me as I was so stressed.

As if life wasn't stressful enough, our village flooded on June 28. Even Lourdes Hospital, a thirty minute car ride away from the Village of Owego, had to be evacuated due to flood waters.

Bill and I worked on medical bills. After a very stressful production of it all, we were okay except for one minor $15 item. Bill kept saying over and over, "This is bad." I told Bill he couldn't keep stressing me like that; to me, $15 was not bad as long as it prolonged my life.

Chapter 24: Letter from the First Lady

I received a reply to my letter from Laura Bush, The White House, Washington DC!

Dear Mrs. Franz,

Thank you for your letter about stem cell research and for telling me about your personal experience. I am delighted to know about your "second chance at life" that resulted from your autologous adult stem cell transplant. Your views on this topic are very much in line with the President's. As he said in a speech on May 25, 2005:

I believe America must pursue the tremendous possibilities of science, and I believe we can do so while still fostering and encouraging respect for human life in all its stages. In the complex debate over embryonic stem cell research, we must remember that real human lives are involved—both the lives of those with diseases that might find cures from this research, and the lives of the embryos that will be destroyed in the process.

President Bush delivered the first ever federal funding for embryonic stem cell research. While the President's policy does not ban, limit, or restrict stem cell research of any kind, it does not provide federal funding for stem cell research that would require the destruction of human embryos.

A tremendous amount of both public and private research is underway in American on embryonic, as well as adult stem cells, and stem cells from umbilical cord blood. Stem cell research involving blood from umbilical cords or adult bone marrow has already led to medical advances and offers enormous potential for many more. Such research never requires the destruct ion of human life. In addition, researchers are exploring way to obtain the same kind of cells now derived from embryos without harming or taking life.

The administration has supported a great deal of ethical

research. About 600 shipments of eligible stem cell lines are already being used by researchers across the country, and over 3,000 more shipments are still available. Federal funding for all forms of stem cell research has increased by more than 80 percent since President Bush took office.

America needs people like you who are interested in the important issues facing our great country. President Bush joins me in sending appreciation for your letter.

With best wishes,
Laura Bush

Chapter 25: Decisions, Treatments and Whatever

I called Laura NP in Syracuse to say I had definitely decided on an adult stem cell transplant. She said it would be covered financially under doctor billings. I'd be on Thalomid for four months which would mean I'd have my transplant in early November. Bill and I discussed our finances and I prayed that we would find favor before God and mankind, especially the insurance company so we had good coverage toward my prescriptions.

I drafted a new letter, entitled "New York State Should Invest in the Right Kind of Stem Cell Research," and mailed copies to politicians and newspapers.

After Mass I looked out my kitchen window and there was Fr. Tom taking a nap on my patio. When Kathy stopped by to visit, she asked Fr. Tom to pray over me. He complied (in tongues) and anointed me with oil. Kathy listened intently to some of the words and she thought Fr. Tom was speaking Greek and names of saints. I was deep in prayer and felt very peaceful.

My reading comforted me: "Go forward unafraid. Face each difficulty as you go towards it. The strength you will require from Me will fortify you."[2]

The reading for the following night was just as sustaining: "Still go forward unafraid. The way will open as you go. It is fear that blocks My way for you. Have no fear. Know that all is well. Trust. Go on in faith and trust. The Way opens as you go forward in firm trust. This is your work. Mine is to cause doors to open as you come to them, not before. More will open as they have in the past so trust, hope and love."[3] I took this to mean my giving presentations on my adult stem cell transplants even while I was going through cancer again was part of God's plan for me. Praise the Lord! What do people do without faith?

Margaret and Cliff Teague stopped by. I haven't seen Margaret since our 1960 high school graduation. She now resided in North Carolina. She was a cancer and heart attack survivor and a strong Christian. Margaret and her husband were going to duplicate my tape to give it a more professional sound.

I had developed a sinus infection and a terrible cough, but Dr. Cooke medicated me for it. Wasn't having cancer enough to battle without my nose, sinuses and throat getting into the act? The steroids were affecting my eyesight which wasn't as sharp due to all the fluid I was retaining. And worst of all, I was growing larger in size almost daily!

Some good news came on my e-mail. I heard from Phil, the medical student I conversed with on the plane. Phil wrote, "I think your story is inspirational and it will always stick with me as I proceed through my medical education and career. Thank you very much for the e-mails. I have read through them and I am also looking forward to searching through the websites to learn more. I have spent a lot of time reading about embryonic stem cells and debating the ethics of such work. After learning this information about adult stem cells it seems that even if embryonic stem cells were a morally sound course of research in their own right (which I don't believe) that it would still be wrong to focus on the research when such a pragmatic alternative exists for helping people. School will start soon. If you would like, I can try to put you in touch with someone about speaking here. If nothing else I look forward to engaging in some interesting discussions with the faculty about this issue. Many thanks and God's richest blessings, Phil."

It was wonderful to get notes like that, because on top of my sinus and coughing issues, my muscles and bones had begun to ache for the first time since my return from Texas. I was off the steroids and the humidity was doing me in.

Thank God for the comfort from my devotional books. "Grace is the distinct mark I set upon My friends. It is the result of living with Me," I read in one. "It is even unobserved by those on whom I bestow it but [visible] to those you meet that have eyes to see. It may be the sign of my sustaining Power, quiet poise, soul unfolding to my Love. Grow daily into my likeness. Do my will as revealed to you and leave the results to Me. Harmonize your mind, body and spirit."[4]

Every day I received cards in the mail but one came that was so beautiful and prayerful that I cried. It was from Marion, whose daughter had passed away. "At times, life's path seems filled with things that make the going rough, And we wish there were a soother road for we feel we've had enough…But, if we pause a moment and remember Who's in charge, The hills that loom ahead of us no longer seem so large, And every rock before us, when we know we're not alone, Becomes, not just a stumbling block, but one more stepping stone. You have overcome so many things, and, every time, you've grown through sheer determination and the wisdom that you've shown. So, as you face this journey, from the moment you begin, Know that God will guide you, and you'll have the strength to win. From the writings of Emily Matthews…..Dear Carol, these words say it all. God Bless you. You are in my prayers, Marion."

There But For the Grace of God

The Lord brought so many decent people into my life that I was truly blessed. I had no fear because I believed I was guided in all I did as I dwelled in the Secret Place of the Most High.

I got on my high horse and sent e-mails to many senators due to embryonic funding bill S5 coming up for vote. Thank God my President said he'd veto it. I wished the public understood how embryonic trials has taken funding from adult stem cell research which has thousands of survivors but needs funding to get more adult stem cell therapies out to the ill.

A priest inspired me today when he stated, "If you trust in God a little you get a little grace. Trust in God with all your heart and grace fills you abundantly."

A friend asked me why people hated President Bush so much. In my opinion, I believe it is because of where the haters are in their Holy Spirit indwelling. Hate is giving in to the enemy and not of the Lord so the haters are being blinded by Satan. Hate does not come from the Lord.

I made several calls to several places and pharmacies to get prescription help after Bill and I spent three hours doing our medical bills. I contacted the Rural Health Network, Office of the Aging, Celegene (manufacturer of Thalomid), Chronic Disease Fund, and the International Myeloma Foundation. I told all these agencies I could not afford my medicines. Our Visa bill was $7,000 which was mostly medicines and doctors bills.

My eyes were bothering me and I had to wear a baseball cap to keep the light out of my eyes. It seemed harder to read as my eyes felt swollen from the steroids, as did my whole body.

I had blood work done at Broome Oncology. Debbie, a social worker, helped me with forms to Celgen for possible help with Thalomid costs. I also filled out forms for help from the Leukemia, Lymphoma and Myeloma Foundation. On my way home I was coughing so badly that I stopped at Dr. Cooke's office. They took me right in. I still had bronchitis which the steroid masked so I was back on antibiotics again. They only charged me $5. Fr. Tom was in our pool when we got home so he stayed for lunch and prayed with me.

President Bush vetoed federally funding embryonic research bill 810 and received a lot of flack. People were so ignorant about adult stems that have helped people and about embryonic stem cells that to my knowledge have helped no one! I e-mailed Maggie and Brenda about their Representatives Castle (Delaware) and DeGette (Colorado) who fought against bill S2754, the Alternative Stem Cell Therapies Enhancement Act, and successfully brought it down by a vote of 273-154, claiming the bill would distract from embryonic stem cell research. The bill would have helped adult stem cell research which included umbilical cord blood research funding. Adult stem cell research is the only stem cell research that had been successful in humans.

A message for me was, "Do not recognize your illness. Each time you speak of it to others, you stabilize it. Claim healing of spirit, mind and body. Then shall you know wholeness."

Whenever I was not so swollen around my eyes, I got on the computer attempting to learn more about multiple myeloma, but all the information I found was very confusing.

Terry and Molly arrived from Georgia. Terry weeded all my flower beds and planted bulbs for me as I was not supposed to put my hands in soil due to the presence of bacteria and fungus.

We attended the Tioga County Relay for Life at Owego Free Academy. I talked to Wendy from the *Pennysaver* whose uncle had a stem cell transplant. I told her to say adult stem cell so people got it right. Embryonic stem cell research, so far, never had a human success story but there are over 400,000 people treated with adult stem cells. At the relay I also talked with Kathy, who is a 1990 adult stem cell transplant survivor of breast cancer,

Five days off steroids and I had more energy and brain function. I had one or two bowel movements daily when off the steroids.

Terry and I watched DVDs from the International Myeloma Foundation that were so informative that she and I wanted to attend a seminar. Terry, Molly, Bill and I went to see Dr. Sheth at Broome Oncology because Lourdes Hospital in Binghamton was not repaired yet from the June flood. My IgA protein level went from 1,505 to 114. Normal is 50-410. Igg went from 491 to 357. Normal Igg is 650-1500. Igm went from 20 to 27. Normal is 60-280. White Blood Count went from 3.3 up to 4.7. Normal is 4.8-10.8. HGB went from 9.2 up to 11 whereas normal is 11.0-15.5. HCT 26.5 was up to 32.4. Normal is 33.0-48.0. Platelets went from 86 up to 135. The normal is 150-450. I weighed 175 pounds which is 35 more than usual. Terry asked good questions of Dr. Sheth and I taped his answers. He said Velcade would be a possible treatment in the future if I ever needed it. I was to get Zometa, a bone strengthener, in four to eight weeks.

I called Sarah and Kathy and told them my good news from Dr. Sheth. I also told them that due to my working with Debbie, the social worker, Celgen offered to give me six months of Thalomid free.

I wrote to Colleen Miner, Ogdensburg Diocese about my good news. She informed me that much interest had been generated for my October presentations in Watertown and Plattsburgh, New York. She also was writing an article for the *North Country Catholic* about the presentations in hope many priests and parishioners would show up.

The girls, Bill and I drove to Malone, New York where we met up with Tyler and Dan at Craig's house. Dan and Craig were in their annual golf tournament with Ty, their nephew, as their caddy. Dan gave me business cards he had made for me that showed my photo, name, address and phone number, and told I am a cancer survivor and adult stem cell transplant recipient. I was thrilled; as these cards would be wonderful to hand out to inform people.

I got weepy too much, ate too much and had difficulty controlling my bladder but I knew it was because of the steroids. I hoped in the Lord for the money to pay for my transplant!

Craig's neighbor was running for a state office so I gave him my card and paperwork on adult stem cell versus embryonic stem cell treatments and research successes. He, like most people, was unaware of the two types of stem cell research.

As I gave the priest at Notre Dame my card after Mass, he informed me that he has read all my articles and encouraged me to keep being an advocate and informing people.

We took Dan, Tyler, Terry and Molly to the airport. When we got home I received a call from Wayne in Kansas asking about adult stem cell therapy for MS and also for breast cancer. I gave him websites, www.stemcellresearch.org and www.clinicaltrials.gov to check out.

Sarah drove me to a chiropractor as my hips ached and my left foot still hurt as it had for the last ten days. Dr. Fluegel sent me to the hospital for an x-ray, after which I returned home. The doctor called 45 minutes later to say the x-ray showed a fifth metatarsal base fracture. He said to get a boot and use a cane. No wonder my foot hurt too much to walk on it when I was in Malone!

Our car had a flat tire, so I called Sandy and she took me to Johnson City to get a foot brace/boot. Insurance covered most of the cost so I only had to pay $39. I had to wear it for six weeks but could shower and sleep without it. I treated Sandy to lunch and when we arrived back at my house she offered us their third car while ours was repaired. We have such caring, helpful friends. We had to have all new tires specially ordered as our car is a Honda Odyssey.

By that time, though, I had been on my foot so long that it really ached. I couldn't even get out of bed, and Bill, who was taking a nap, didn't hear me calling him. I phoned Joan who knocked at the door to awaken Bill. She got me an ice bag for my sore ankle and visited with me. At six o'clock when I got hungry, I called Bill on the cell phone to our house phone to fix me supper. He heard my voice on the answering machine and came in to the bedroom. I dutifully stayed off my foot except for bathroom breaks and retrieving ice.

"Love and care and pray. Never feel helpless to aid those I love. I am their help. As I obey Christ and follow His teaching in my daily life, I will bring that help into operation. So, if I desire to be used to save another, turn up my own life, as far as I can, make it all that it should be. Let my influence for Jesus extend further and further. Let Love be my balm for all ills."[5]

I was not feeling well enough to go to Mass as I was incredibly tired. I talked, cried and hugged Bill, sharing my feelings of being alone in this second cancer as I lacked companionship and felt left out.

I received an e-mail from Laura at Upstate that said I should call Dr. Sheth about the fluid in my face and also see an eye doctor.

Dr. Sheth said my blood work was better than most people working at the hospital. White blood count normal, 5.1, HCT 12 & normal, platelets 167, first normal in 3 years, and my red blood count is 37.1 and normal. Due to my puffy face he was giving me less dexamethansone steroid. I should take it eight days a month instead of twelve. I asked why I was so tired and he said that the meds and lack of exercise were responsible. Since I still had the boot on my foot, I needed to do upper body weights and stretches. I was to receive Zometa for my bones.

Dr. Williams checked my eyes and explained how the steroid was responsible for the fluid buildup in my body, head and eye area. Thalomid was a drug used for some eye problems and he was very familiar with it.

I went to Broome Oncology for my Zometa infusion and also picked up the free Thalomid for the month. Mercifully, I received word from the Leukemia, Lymphoma and Myeloma Foundation which said I had been approved for $500 in aid. Praise the Lord!

Since I was now feeling a bit better, Bill dropped me off for this month's Charismatic Healing Mass. The St. John's music group provided the music and they were wonderful as usual. Fr. Boniface anointed each of the people there with oil. Prayers were said in tongues as Fr. Boniface roamed the congregation claiming healings for various diseases. I claimed those for Pat and Brenda as well as Joan and myself. When Fr. Boniface told us to touch our affected parts of our bodies, I touched myself from feet to shoulders to head. Marti came behind me, laid her hands on my shoulders and prayed over me. My whole body was so heated and I could feel the Holy Spirit working. When Marti touched me I could feel such tremendous heat from her hand. Joan and I were both very heated. Fr. Boniface asked for prayers for safety because priests are being killed in Africa where he was heading for a while. He told me he prayed for me and told his people in Africa of my positive spirit. Fr. Watts said to keep writing my book.

Bill then dropped me off at Curves and I worked on my upper body for about forty-five minutes. That same evening, Bill and I attended a Lion's Club meeting at Donoli's Restaurant. I spoke on stem cell research, my experience, explained cloning and discussed Congress's voting record on three bills, two of which passed. Congress voted for saving of cord blood, voted against funding for adult and ethical embryonic stem cell research and just voted for funding of embryonic stem cell research.

At Sunday Mass with Fr. Boniface presiding, I received the Lord and kept him on my tongue to anoint my tongue and speech. Tears came to my eyes just knowing that Jesus was physically in me. The sermon was about going to the Word of God instead of TV and media for direction and values.

I decided to fast and pray for the parental knowledge bill the Democrats were stalling in Washington, DC. If this bill passed, a minor girl could be taken across state lines to get an abortion without her parents' consent or knowledge. To me that's kidnapping! I get so frustrated over people who worry about the poor, money and yet don't seem to care about the destruction of unborn children or embryos.

Diane called to see if I needed any grocery shopping done. Bless her heart. Two weeks ago she drove me to her beauty shop, cut my hair, wheeled me around in a wheelchair at the grocery store, brought me home and put my groceries in the cupboard for me. Diane was being Christ to me.

As a grandma of faith, I felt prompted by the Holy Spirit when I sent Ty a birthday card and wrote the following:

> "We were born to know, love and serve God in this world and the next, Heaven. We are made of body, soul and spirit. To keep balanced physically, mentally and spiritually is not easy. It is easier to work out, learn in school, but often the spiritual can be neglected. Take the values of God, not the World, to live by. The World can lead many astray. Desire and pray for the Wisdom of God which is meant to activate your mental talents… understanding, reason, and peace. God created the Mass so that He could come to us. As we gather to celebrate the Eucharist, we confess our sins and our need for God's mercy. "This softens our hearts so the Word of God, Bible readings, can take root in us. We profess our faith with the creed. We pray for others and lift our hearts in praise and thanksgiving.
>
> Through the actions of the Holy Spirit, bread and wine are transformed into Jesus and we receive Him in communion. John 6:53-58 says: "If you do not eat the flesh of the Son of Man and drink His blood you will not have life within you." This is the basis of the Catholic Church which has passed down from the Lord and apostles at the Last Supper.
>
> Ty, I love you so much and desire for you the peace, inner strength and faith that sustain me. My prayer for all our family,

which includes your dad, is a deep abiding faith. I realize this is unusual to receive a note as this on your 18th birthday but I felt the need to write you. Keep it and read it each year as you age,

Love and hugs,
Grandma

I was back on Dex and really, really sleepy so I went back to bed even though it was mid-morning. Jane, who is a retired nurse, called to say that my adult stem cell transplant should go smoother this time around because I was in better condition. It helped to have such a positive talk.

Bill and I attended a Leukemia, Lymphoma and Myeloma support group meeting in Endicott, NY. Ray, Mary Lou Robinson and I were first-timers and the three of us all suffered with multiple myeloma. Others there had different diseases. Ray didn't have enough cells for transplant but meds are helping him as was Zometa. Mary Lou had an adult stem cell transplant for myeloma and was also was a breast cancer survivor. Comparing my situation to others I met, I felt as though I was in good enough shape for another transplant.

Once I got home, though, I had gut pain, my head filled with sounds like hundreds of insects, my eyes would not focus, I had no energy and I wanted to cry. I offered it up to God. The pain in my gut spread to my legs and feet, and I felt weak and strange all over. I concluded it was the steroid, although this hadn't happened to me before. Petie called to invite me to lunch. She prayed over the phone with me and I got better and the pain went away.

I received a letter from Yvonne in England which always boosted my spirits. "Dear Carol and Bill, Thank you for the details of your treatment. It gives us a target for prayer. Last night I woke in the night with a prayer burden for you. I also prayed this a.m. and of course we remembered you at our group meeting. You are doing well with your crusade informing folks about the virtues and successes of adult stem cell transplants. Hang in there, Carol -- your situation must add weight to your words, and your sincerity is clear to see. God bless you and yours richly, may He hold you up and give you his strength, peace and comfort."

Mike Latona of the Rochester Diocese *Catholic Courier* interviewed me on September 11 concerning my experience with adult stem cells. I wasn't feeling my best. I was so tired that I had urine and blood work testing done, as well as a mammogram and Pap smear. Dr. Miller told me I had vaginal atrophy which made intercourse painful. My low platelet counts precluded intercourse, anyway, due to the likelihood of internal bleeding. My spirit perked up when Dr. Carol Miller told me she loved my positive, upbeat attitude and my multi-colored polish on my toes.

On my return home I called Laura at Upstate Medical in Syracuse and she answered questions I had concerning the adult stem cell transplant. Recovery times would be two to six months. Survival rate was 98%. The cost of the transplant would be $84,000. IgA capa B was the form of multiple myeloma I had. Dex steroid and thalidomide would just buy me time before a transplant. I must go off the drugs a while before the transplant procedure was done. I reread the stem cell transplant book from Upstate Medical. All the side effects listed sounded terrible but Laura NP sounded so positive, and a 98% survival rate sounded good as well.

I was late for my appointment with Dr. Sheth at Broome Oncology, but it turned out to be a good thing as they were backed up thirty patients. My blood IgA was 57, red 3.20L, HGB 11.2L, HCT 33.2L and platelets 157. Dr. Sheth wanted my jaw pain checked out by a dentist before I could receive anymore Zometa.

Bill and I went from Syracuse to Clayton, New York on the St. Lawrence River and stayed with Mary Lou and Al Seymour. Mary Lou drove me in our car to Immaculate Heart Central School in Watertown where I spoke at the Life and Family Conference of the Ogdensburg Diocese on September 19 and 20, 2007. There were about 100 junior and senior year high school students plus many priests and other adults. Kathy Gallagher of the NYS Catholic Conference gave a presentation on cloning and stem cell research after which I told my personal story. We both answered questions from the audience. I received a BOGO wine set. BOGO had adult stem cell information on the bottle as well as on the packing, and a percentage of each sale went to adult stem cell research. A woman told me she and her prayer group would pray for me. She was in awe that I would be witnessing while I was going through cancer treatments. I also was wearing that lovely boot on my broken foot!

Mary Lou and I returned to her place and then Bill and I drove on to Malone, New York to stay overnight at our son's home. The next day, Craig, Bill and I left Malone, traveling to St. Peter's Church in Plattsburgh where Craig videotaped my presentation. I met several priests, an interdenominational Protestant pastor, nurses, nuns and lay people who asked many questions. This was the first time Craig had heard my presentation.

I had to return to Owego right away as a Rochester *Catholic Courier* photographer named Mike was coming to take photos of me for an article in the *Courier*. He spent about an hour taking many photo shots.

What a week! I went to see Dr. Cooke because my foot was still swollen. He was impressed with my blood work as I showed him a copy I carried with me. His nurse made a copy for his office. The blood work also showed that my kidney functions were good as well.

I caught up on 73 e-mails even though my bones ached and my muscles were cramped. It was my second night without Thalomid. I lost some fluid but no weight according to the scales. I cried when I received communion at Mass as my Lord was so personal to me.

Again I was at Broome Oncology for blood work. I also met with Dr. James DeSantis, a dental surgeon, who examined my jaw and said I had tendonitis in my face near my cheek bones that could affect the muscles near my hairline parallel to my eyes. He instructed me to use warm compresses, massage and Tylenol. Thank God I did not have jaw-death from Zometa!

I heard from Colleen Miner on the Life and Family Conference. Father Mark told her that many students talked with him following my testimony and said how cool it was to actually meet someone who used the therapy that Kathy Gallagher talked about. Colleen had people in Plattsburgh comment about how interesting it was to learn about adult stem cell treatment and then to meet someone who benefited from it. She thanked me for my bravery and willingness to share. I wrote back to her that my son, husband and the friends who attended were all impressed by the folder handouts, the food and the items on display. I was so glad my folder had a pen with the little ten week fetus-size feet imprinted on it. That will bring comments whenever I let folks use my pen in my travels. I plan on taking the pen to Syracuse with me in the transplant unit.

Terry called to say that her class received and discussed a booklet on dealing with stress. She reminded me that when she was stressed I told her to "count her blessings" and she did. I spoon-fed her spiritual directions and Bible verses often.

Chapter 26: Whoops!

I met with Dr. Gentile at the ROC (Regional Oncology Center) at the Syracuse Upstate Medical Hospital. She was pleased with my blood and protein counts. I would skip a stay in the hospital for heavy chemo and go right to admittance for transplant. When in the hospital I would get a catheter installed in my chest. My tests from Broome Oncology showed no multiple myeloma in my urine, or in my bones. My bone density survey showed just arthritis and demineralization (in other words, my bones were thinning). Bone marrow showed 61% cancer cells so I would have another bone marrow tap. I would also receive no Zometa because my bones looked so good. A flu shot would be needed after I had the bone marrow biopsy done. I needed to receive immunization shots one year after transplant. My boot must be off my foot before I could have the transplant. I asked and was told that adult stem cells do not cause cancer. Dr. Gentile did the bone marrow biopsy tap and it was the least painful I have ever had.

However, my path to transplant hit a small bump. After the bone marrow tap, as I got off the table I became dizzy. I sat in a chair and the nurse called for Dr. Gentile. Dr. Gentile asked me questions and for a while all I could say was abba, abba. That meant Father God! She sent me immediately for a MRI x-ray as soon as I recovered, which took about five minutes. The MRI showed constricted blood vessels in my brain. The doctor explained that I had a TIA or transient ischemic attack, and was told I had small vessel ischemic disease. This slowed blood flow. My blood pressure was 184 over 101 after the TIA but then gradually dropped back to normal. I was told to take a baby aspirin every evening, and I had to see a neurologist before I could have the transplant.

When we left the hospital at 5:00 PM, we stopped at Dinosaur BBQ Biker Restaurant for supper as we had missed lunch. I put my right leg out of the car and then attempted to lift my casted left foot out and I heard sounds from my back. When I tried to put weight on my legs, my knee just buckled from the pain and I couldn't walk or stand. The pain was more intense that I usually have with biopsies. Bill didn't want to return to the Syracuse hospital so I called to "report" problems as the paperwork had requested. I got a doctor who said to go to an emergency room. Bill wanted to drive to an ER nearer to home, so we bought burgers at Wendy's and ate them in car as we drove the 90 miles on Route 81 home. Lourdes' emergency room was packed so we went to Wilson Hospital where, after obtaining a wheelchair, he took me into reception. We were the second name on the list but the last one to be seen, and we got out of there at 2:00 AM.

I had two x-rays which showed old lesions only -- nothing broken or dislocated. Bill didn't think he could drive home as he was so tired but the cold outdoor air revived him. He and I had clashed earlier in the day, as he didn't like my questioning the doctor so much when he was so tired and hungry. I kept my mouth shut at first but when he kept complaining about his health, I said I'd gladly let him have my cancer. After my slight seizure he treated me so sweetly. I think he got scared.

The day after all the excitement, I rested my sore biopsy spot and my foot. I called Dr. Cooke to make an appointment, as he had to see me before he could set me up with a neurologist. Laura Tormey NP called from Syracuse to say my bone marrow biopsy showed the cancer went from 61.5% down to 6%. Praise the Lord!

Sadly, I found out my cousin's wife, Traci Gibson, died. Traci fought her battle with breast cancer to the very end. Traci's Hope, a fund raiser to help breast cancer patients, would go on even though she was gone. She so much wanted to help others. There would always be a celebration of Traci Shiner Gibson's life.

On October 5, I was allowed to remove the bandage from my biopsy. It was very dried but bloodier than ever before. I saw Dr. Cooke who had talked with Dr. Gentile. They agreed on an ultrasound of my neck (a stress ECHO carotid duplex), an ECHO cardiogram and a 24-hour heart halter monitor. If all was normal I wouldn't have to see a neurologist. I was instructed to take a regular aspirin, not a baby aspirin. In one week I would get my foot x-rayed.

Several people called to tell me my photo was on the cover of the Rochester *Catholic Courier* and that a three-page article was inside the *Courier*. A couple of people called to say my photo and the story of my presentations in Watertown and Plattsburgh were in the North Country, Ogdensburg Diocese newspaper. How nice it was to have people keep me informed. There are so many good, caring people in this world who don't ask for any attention but are just Christ-like to others.

I read in Psalm 121.8 "The Lord shall preserve thy going out and thy coming in from this time forth and even for evermore." I took this to mean that all my movements, my goings and comings are controlled by God. Every visit or speech on adult stem cells that I have ever given or will ever give is blessed by God. There is a blessing on all I do, on every interview – and an assurance that every meeting is not a chance meeting, but planned by my

There But For the Grace of God

God. All blessed and not only now, in the hour of any difficulty, but from this time forth and forevermore. I believe I am led by the Spirit, a proof of Sonship. What a heritage! I am an heir of God and a joint heir with Christ, so that that if I suffer with Him I may also be glorified with Him

So my suffering had its purpose. It was proof of Sonship. It led to perfection of character (the being glorified) and to Union with God too. Think of, and dwell upon, the rapture of this. What comfort this gave me!

Art gave me a booklet that included this passage: "Sin brought a curse on the earth and its people (Genesis 3:15-24). This curse included sin and death. Suffering awakens compassion. We can use suffering as an opportunity to serve God by helping others, to trust God in spite of our difficulties and to grown in our faith in Him. Because we are a social race, our lives are intertwined so we sometimes suffer when the sins or foolishness of others spreads trouble. Our response to suffering shows our caliber of humanity." Wow! This sure puts what I had been going through in perspective.

The Lord kept feeding me spiritual nourishment, such as these words from Fr. Frank Pavone of Priests for Life. "Defend life......Unborns are innocents put to death. Those who die in war are defending life. Those who die because of the death penalty are not innocents who never had a chance to live. Be a Catholic first then a political party member second. Remember the party matters. When you vote for someone in a party, even if they are pro-life and the party isn't, the party platform will reign. A question to ask a candidate is: if your party supports abortion, would you take a stand and disagree? Find out [each] party's policies and principals as they differ." I remembered this information when I was looking at whom to vote for.

I went to Lourdes Hospital in Binghamton for the ultrasound on my neck, the echocardiogram of my heart and a twenty-four hour heart monitor. The echocardiogram technician said, "You seem to have trouble breathing," but I said, "No. Only a couple times when on my Thalomid and Dex, but not now." I had the x-rays and went shopping with Bill.

The next day, I'd had very little sleep due to the heart monitor. Bill and I drove to Lourdes where they unhooked me, and we went home. I received a phone call from an RN at United Healthcare. She called to see if I was in the hospital for my transplant. She said my transplant has been approved by UH insurance. She knew very little about adult stem cell research and therapies so I explained some stuff to her. She was amazed!

In mid-October, we drove to Rochester during a snow storm, where Bill and I attended an Adult Stem Cell Initiative program featuring David A. Prentice, Ph.D., Senior Fellow for Life Sciences at the Family Research Council and Center for Life and Bioethics. This was held at the Rochester Academy of Medicine. I wore my lime green shirt that said Adult Stem Cell

Transplant Survivor and many recognized me from the picture and article in the Rochester Diocese *Catholic Courier*. Dr. Prentice asked me to send my story to be included on www.stemcellresearch.org. We stayed for the reception where people asked Bill and me lots of questions. I met a few people who were unable to use Thalomid due to side effects. I was so blessed that my body tolerated it. We got back home about midnight as it is a three hour car ride. I was so energized I was up until 3 AM.

Jane called me from Vegas. She had bought her first Bible and asked me how to look up things in it. She had been reading the *Daily Word* that I sent her as a gift. I told her that when I came to Las Vegas we would do a Bible study together. I worked via computer as I had lots of e-mails to answer. I read that to break into spontaneous songs of praise and prayer, a Christian has to be vibrant and lively. I do that, so I must be vibrant and lively!

I wondered how many cancer patients with a broken bone in their foot exercise like I did five days a week at Curves. I bet not many. I stopped at the Board of Elections to vote and Mary Jane Robie was there to vote as well. Later on she asked me, "How did you know who to vote for?" I said, "It was easy. I just voted for the pro-life candidates because without life a person has nothing." I spoke to a Democrat worker in the hallway and asked her what could be done to get the Democrat Party's attention concerning adult stem cell research versus embryonic. I told her how so many of them on the Hill in Washington, DC ignored me. She was sad and serious and said there seemed to be nothing we could do.

But that's just not in my vocabulary!

Chapter 27: Hurry up Already

Finally, half-way through the month of October, my foot was healed. Dr. Cooke said all my other tests and heart monitor were normal and the boot came off my foot. I drove for the first time in ten weeks and attended St. Patrick's Church Charismatic Healing Mass. I hung a copy of my interview in the *Catholic Courier* on the bulletin board at church. The next day I drove myself to Curves for exercise. My friends and Bill no longer had to be my drivers. I heard back positive comments from some of the pro-life politicians I contacted.

We had such cold weather in Owego that my hands were sore and stiff and the skin on them cracked as well. I dislike winter and winter doesn't like me much either!

I received a letter from someone I don't know, but whom Bill knew growing up on the Flats section of Owego. Adrian wrote on October 17, 2006:

"Dear Carol,

A few years ago I was with my 1958 OFA Reunion at the Parkview Restaurant. You and Bill were there. Bill and I attended St. Pat's School and OFA, and we were 'Flat Rats.' Bill was one year ahead of me in school. He came over to talk with me. I had not seen Bill for a ton of years. When he told me that you had adult stem cell treatment, I was absolutely stunned. Of course, I had seen bits and pieces on TV and read a little about them here and there, but until then I thought stem cell treatment was a thing of the future. Of course I was delighted for you and your family. Since then whenever I visit Mom in Candor, New York, I read over her old papers that she saves for me, and there often is a piece written by you about adult stem cells.

You are doing a terrific job letting us know your first hope experience. Nonetheless, not too long ago I was asking myself what happens when a disease returns after treatment. Your article in the Rochester *Catholic Courier* answered that question. I am tickled that you will try again. Anyone that would marry someone from Owego's Flats deserves a carefree and long, long life. Please continue to educate us Flat Rats. Respectfully, Adrian."

I was phoned by a Republican Party woman asking for a donation. I told her I had a $84,000 adult stem cell transplant coming up and couldn't send any money. She said that she would add me to her prayer list and told me to read the 91st Psalm every day. I thanked her for sharing her faith.

I received a letter from a man troubled about his job and I was led by the Spirit to respond, "I understand your feelings but don't let your feelings rule your mind. I know you probably don't want to read this but you need to take your problems to the Lord and especially develop more of a relationship with Him. We just don't go to Him with problems but also go to Him in praise and worship. In my own experience, especially in the last four months, my worshipping and taking just a few minutes to read scripture or say a rosary have filled me with such blessed peace and guided me in my actions.

"Don't let that fallen angel, Satan, fill your mind with negative feelings and thoughts about yourself. You are a child of God and a unique individual who is a blessing to all who know you. When I have hard times I offer my struggles up to the Lord in intercession for others such as yourself or our military. Love is a decision we make as is working and worshipping. We decide to do them even though we don't feel like it. Feelings are not right or wrong -- they just are -- but they don't decide who and what we are or what we do. If I let feelings rule me, I'd stay in bed all day reading books or watching TV. Love, Carol."

I attended Saturday night Mass in a pink and black felt poodle skirt complete with a crinoline, a 50s pink shell and black top, socks with poodles on them, Bill's class ring around my neck on a chain, white sneakers (no longer had white buck shoes) and my OFA wool cheerleading jacket. After Mass in the church hall there was a 50s murder mystery dinner show. I got a lot of strange looks during Mass but I fit right in at the dinner show. We had a great time and even danced a few dances. My clothes were uncomfortable because of all the weight gain from my medicines but I persevered.

Chapter 28: Here I Go, Ready or Not

Laura, my NP from Upstate Medical in Syracuse e-mailed me to let me know that Monday, October 30 was my admittance date at the hospital. I e-mailed family and friends to let them know my transplant was set to go. I received several e-mails and phone calls of encouragement. Diane cut off my hair, getting me ready for my hospital stay and hair fall-out. Karen from the Coburn Free Library sent three books for me to take to the hospital with me. I believed my faith level was good and I still worked out at Curves daily until I left for the hospital. My bags were packed and I was eager to get started.

I awoke on October 25 aching in my bones, and I felt so poorly I cried. Marion Davis called me, and she told me that she meant to call someone else but her mistake was part of God's plan and comforted me. She added my name to the church's prayer list. Sarah and Sue Ann called while I was still crying and also prayed for me.

The following day, I was still aching, especially my previously broken foot. It must be the stinky New York weather, Praise the Lord. At Curves today, a woman said she was putting me on the Presbyterian prayer chain. Agnes, a woman that used to work with my mom at the EJ Shoe Factory in the 1940s, called to say she was praying with me.

I also received a note from Sandy Solomon. "Although our paths have not crossed, I think of you often and you remain on my prayer list. I just want you to know that I see your beautiful radiance as the presence of the Holy Spirit within and surrounding you. Your gentleness, your words and your life give glory to our Lord that more might believe. You are special, Carol, and I am just one more person who believes that. May you continue to experience His peace and love. God bless, Sandy S."

I am on my third day of aching like a son of a gun thanks to the good old cold weather. I must remember that Jesus shared our sufferings and showed us the way. Suffering makes you grateful, kind and more loving. Suffering is valued by God. Suffering purifies us and not just physical suffering. We grow in virtue, growth of our soul and suffering participates in our being the image of Jesus. Suffering was for my own good and been good for me.

Pete Premock called from Cape Cod and put Nan on the phone who asked questions about adult stem cell transplants for multiple myeloma. Nan's friend is going to Upstate Medical for a transplant in November.

Random thoughts kept coming to me. I didn't know if I read them somewhere or if it was the Holy Spirit. People suffering and not healed are being sanctified for Heaven. Everything I do and say depends on my faith level. God's will be done. Sometimes we heal others by the benefit of our pain. You don't need yourself as much as you need God. Offer suffering up for others. I do know Cardinal Newman said, "Error may flourish for a time but truth will prevail in the end." Awesome thoughts for me to contemplate!

October 29 was my last Sunday home before admission to the hospital. It was very cold with a light snow and a wind advisory in effect. Bill brought me home communion from church, and it was a special moment of union with the Lord before my time of trial.

Chapter 29: Adult Stem Cell Transplant #2

I arrived at Upstate Medical at 10 AM on October 30. After registering, I went directly to radiology and was kept in the prep room for two hours. A nurse practitioner talked to me about positive thinking and explained how I could tell my body to be well. While I was in a bed in the hallway outside the radiation room, a man in scrubs passed by, patted me gently on my head and smiled. Another female nurse past by and patted my shoulder. Their compassion meant much to me and was a sign to me that the Lord was with me.

Finally I was taken into the room, put under a tent, prepped with an iodine wash on my skin and had a tri-fusion catheter installed. An ultrasound of my vein on the right side of neck, my oxygen levels, and blood pressure were checked throughout the procedure. A nurse laughed and talked with me. One of our topics was margarita consumption. None of those working on me had knowledge of adult stem cell therapies nor the 400,000 humans treated using adult stem cells. They seemed quite enthused as I explained the failures of embryonic stem cell treatments. Leave it to me to be educating those working on my body.

A nurse, Robin, took me to my room, switched me from a bed to a wheelchair and off we went to have my lungs x-rayed. I was told me they do this to check that the port was in the correct place and that there were no nicks in other places like my lungs.

I was given Vancomysin, an antibiotic, and Cumadin, which prevented blood clots forming. I had an infusion of saline solution and chemo Melphalan and also potassium as it was low. (I would also be taking Protonix in the evening with a steroid, Decadron.) The nurse checked my lungs by having me take breaths four times. Then I was given Acyclovir which prevents herpes, shingles, and brain infections.

Dr. Gentile came in twice to see me. She did the "lung thing," checked me over and talked to my nurses about my medication intolerances. I received an anti-nausea infusion, Kytril. My neck felt tender and I was bleeding a little. My skin was very dry. My pain was gone due to the medication at the port insert site.

At 4 PM I received my only chemo treatment which was fifteen minutes of intense chemo.

I was awakened several times in the night (not a surprise) to replace each potassium bag until I'd received six bags total. Every time the machine beeped, Bill could hear it as he was sleeping on a chair/bed in my room. He changed from day clothes to sweats outfit, used the bathroom down the hall near the elevators and stayed the night with me.

On October 31 my breakfast was served at 8 AM as well as Vancomysin and Acyclovir. My nurses wore Halloween buttons on their scrubs. I wore a Vote Pro-Life button on my robe!

I walked in the hall way a lot (Bill said miles) until my left foot ached where it had been broken. I showered. The room was cleaned. Bill napped. I was feeling normal but didn't sleep much so I ordered an Ambien to take at night.

I had two messages on cell phone that Bill slept through. One was from Kathy and the other was from Terry. I called Kathy at work and gave her my room number, room phone number and the address of the hospital. I left Terry a message with the same information. I asked Bill to e-mail folks.

After a lunch of meatloaf, mashed potatoes, beans and a fruit cup, Robin, my main nurse, took my vitals. We discussed adult stem cell research. I told her facts and showed her information that I had brought to the hospital with me. She made copies of the information and was going to tell her mom to vote for stem cell research using adult stem cells, not embryonic. Democrats are pushing embryonic and Republicans are pushing the adult.

Kevin, a Jesuit novice, visited Bill and I and we received communion. Kevin prayed a beautiful prayer and we said the Our Father together. Kevin told us he had talked to five couples today married over forty-five years and how happy that made him. He was Upstate Medical's Catholic Chaplin on Tuesdays and Thursdays. Mass was at noon on weekdays and at 4 AM on Saturday. Bill made Kevin copies of the 72 therapies presently in use employing adult stem cells versus zero using embryonic therapies. I was wearing my Vote Pro-Life pin on robe so all could see it right through Election Day.

I received cards and phone calls. I called Brenda in Colorado and Craig to tell them that November first was the big day.

Nurse Debbie showed up dressed as "Nurse Betty." We laughed and she even sat down and visited, but stem cell research never came up. She gave me Kytril anti-nausea drip and Decadron. I was going out for walk in the hallway around 3 PM, but nurses were discussing patients so I had to wait in my room until the shift change. At 6 PM I tried for a nap but it was really short; at 6:30 a nurse came to collect my food tray. Bill left at 7 PM to spend the night at the Seymour's.

Before retiring for the night, I called my sister Sue in Florida. She told me her friends said a rosary for me at their meetings and one of her friends read The Rochester Diocese *Catholic Courier* to the group, many of whom didn't know about the success of adult stem cell transplants. Again my "rag-tag army" was spreading the word of hope and health with adult stem cells.

"Nurse Betty" came in to tuck me in for the night; that costume cheered us both up and got us laughing. On a more serious note, we talked about stem cell research, voting and Michael J. Fox, who didn't speak about the wonders of adult stem cell clinical trials for Parkinson's. Then Debbie gave me my five bedtime pills: two for herpes virus protection, Protonix, a blood thinner, and Tylenol to help me sleep.

I was awakened at 4:30 AM for complete blood work. It turns out I weighed 178 pounds. My lungs checked out well and my blood pressure was good. I was lying on my rosary when I awoke so I started saying the Glorious Mysteries before and after, pausing only for the above work by the nurse. Nurse Debbie was always so cheerful, and laughter is such good medicine! Debbie explained how chemo killed all cells swimming around for a few hours, so hopefully all the cancer cells were caught. My blood counts were WBC (white blood count) 4.1, HCT (red blood count) 29.7 and PLT (platelet blood count) 112. Debbie also explained that even after transplant, my cells would continue to fall for a couple days before the counts started going up except for the white which would continue to fall.

I had breakfast of grape juice and Decadron. Whoopee!

Nurse Kitty introduced herself, but I remembered her (as I had Debbie) from my last transplant visit at Syracuse. I had three bags hanging off this thing next to my bed. They contained potassium, saline, 5% dextrose and saline and flush saline.

Bill was emotionally drained by the stress of my treatments, and he slept a lot; he was actually sleeping at the hospital when I received my adult stem cell transplant. This time it was only 2 minus days instead of 5 minus for my first transplant. I have three birthdates now; April 14, 1942, May 20, 2003 and November 1, 2006. I hoped I'd get cards for at least one of them.

At 8:45 AM, Kitty and Dr. Gentile put the syringe with my adult stem cells in the catheter in my chest. My stem cells were from those harvested in 2003, frozen and stored. Dr. Gentile said my cells were very rich. I experienced no side effects such as hot flashes. One vial was used and it took only fifteen minutes as I watched. I still had one vial left stored at Syracuse Hospital. The cells traveled to the bones, set themselves, and dissipated the solution that froze the cells. By that time, the chemo was out of the blood stream in other cells which would be eliminated. The new cells wouldn't be attacked by the chemo. The counts in the chemo-infused blood would drop down, and the new cells haven't set themselves yet to produce new cells. The drug to dissipate the solution caused many potty trips.

I was given Vancomysin for protection and Kytril to reduce nausea.

Around 10 AM, a Lutheran chaplain named Deacon Madeline came in, and we discussed adult stem cells positively. She had a good understanding of the embryonic versus adult stem cell issue. We prayed for voter wisdom on life issues such as adult stem cell research. She said I looked wonderful as most times her patients have layers of skin missing and looked terrible.

When Bill left for lunch in the cafeteria, I had a bowl of soup and watched Catholic Mass on TV as it was All Saints Day. I slept for ten minutes until Nurse Donna brought me in two Tylenol and my Acyclovir.

A little after three, Bill left for home as he had a ninety minute car ride and didn't feel well. He promised to call our sons and tell them how the transplant went.

I had hospital pizza for supper and it was really good. Food was separately made in hospital kitchen and delivered first to the transplant floor. In addition to the pizza, I had grape juice and ginger ale mixed and half a Dixie cup of strawberry ice cream. I was on a neutropenic diet, which is for people with weakened immune systems..

I walked the hallway for twenty minutes to keep my lungs clear.

The tape used on my chest to hold the covering over the catheter was itchy and the skin was red so Nurse Marcia changed the bandage. It really hurt and the iodine stung slightly in the port hole opening. Of course, I showed Nurse Marcia my list of 72 adult stem cell therapies, and told her how adult stem cell treatments had helped patients with diagnoses as diverse as spinal cord injuries and blocked arteries.

I was feeling nauseous so took an Adavan. My nausea aside, I took it as a sign from God that I received my new life's blood on All Saints Day.

I was awakened from sound sleep several times in the night but went right back to sleep until 6:30 AM. Then I awoke with a stuffy nose, achy head and sticky eyes like I was getting a cold. I used nasal spray and eye drops. My ears were plugged, my nose was runny and I coughed.

My blood counts showed my blood was lacking calcium so I was given two bags of calcium electrolytes, six bags of potassium electrolytes which helped the way my heart beat, and Kytril to prevent nausea. I had French toast with syrup, bacon and tea, oatmeal with brown sugar and milk, and cranberry juice for breakfast. I took folic acid pills, a multivitamin (including K), and Acyclovir.

Pat brought communion to me and we talked.

Dr. Gentile told me my port-hole skin had tears so a new type of dressing was needed. I cried as it was so painful to remove the old dressing due to the glue and tape used to hold the gauze on. The changed dressing now has a window and not clorhexidine.

Kevin, a novice from Boston currently at Lemoyne, read the Magnificate to me and we prayed a Hail Mary. He said when I fall asleep praying, graces still flow to me and my intentions. I wept after he left because I was so grateful to my Lord for being with me and sending so many people of faith to me.

Bill called. He contacted several people and listened to numerous phone messages concerning me. He still wasn't feeling well but planned on coming up for the weekend.

For lunch, I had half a cheeseburger, beef soup, prune juice, tea and a chocolate chip cookie.

The noon service on TV was an interfaith service led by a Buddhist. That was my first!

Dan called at 1PM and I cried. He has been my blessing in my aging years. I walked a third of a mile and read cards I received in the mail. Sue forgot to put my name on the front of the card so it went to the Stem Cell Ward and Lab. When they opened it and saw Carol written inside the card they sent it up to the Transplant Unit.

I phoned St. Patrick's Church and asked that our 46th wedding anniversary be remembered in prayer petitions on November 26.

I feel very drowsy and received more IVs of potassium and Acyclovir. Nurse Marcia gave me Lasix which took fluids out of me as I was too filled with sodium saline and gained weight due to the fluid. My blood pressure was down due to the Lasix.

At 8 PM, I received Protonix, Acyclovir and a blood thinner. But I couldn't sleep, and at midnight I was given Ambien, a sleeping aid, and I slept well until I was awakened at 4 AM for blood work. I then slept until 7 AM.

The next day, my blood counts were WBC 1.6, HCT 29.6 and PLT 85. The white and platelets fell but the red improved slightly. My blood pressure was down due to the Lasix eliminating fluids.

Nurse Kitty explained that they have to try to get the covering off the port without hurting my skin. She did a great job bandaging the port while I was talking to Bill on the phone.

I also loved my visits from Evelyn, the hospital cleaning lady, who said she loved to talk about God all day, every day. My first time in here we discussed the Lord a lot. I remember she was struggling and had many questions for me about God, although three years later I couldn't recall the details of those early conversations.

At 8:30 AM the menu planner came in coughing and touching things that I touch. People who work in hospitals shouldn't be spreading disease. This may have upset me so much because I was on a hormone roll, but I cried. I walked another half hour in the hallway, which brought me peace. Dr.

Gentile stopped in and said she was getting eye drops for me and also told me my bone aches are from past breaks.

Louise Maser, a Eucharistic Minister, prayed for me and gave me communion. I explained the difference between adult and embryonic stem cell research, and she prayed for my life and ministry. It was great being able to share my faith with her, and she with me.

I listened to a tape by MariJohn's which contained the phrase "returning to the faith of my mother and God of my father" which brought to mind my parents and how much I missed them. After a short nap, I listened to Sarah's Gospel music tape while eating my lunch of baked fish, spinach and tea. The noon Mass was said by Fr. Innocent from Nigeria.

Sarah Hall and Sally Martin spent two hours with me. Sarah gave me a Chaplet of St. Michael, the Archangel. I also got lots of cards.

I received a wrong number from a Mineola woman calling her aunt who was a patient in the hospital. I told the woman I had an adult stem cell transplant that gave me my life back. She got excited. I repeated the words "adult stem cell transplant." I wished I had said "not embryonic" so I prayed the Lord help her understand what I said.

My supper was pot roast, green beans, mashed potatoes, tea and a chocolate chip cookie which I ate while listening to the Christian music tape Sarah made for me. After dinner I walked the hall. I would do three turns a minute and 60 turns is a mile. They wanted me to walk three miles. I didn't think I could do that in twenty-five minutes but maybe I could do two miles.

After my shower I was bandaged up again; they put Bactracin ointment on my skin to heal it. It helps prevent infection in minor cuts, scrapes, burns and rashes. I was given more Vancomysin, an antibiotic, and then went to sleep.

Dr. Gentile checked me and prescribed a different nausea pill because the other one I was taking made me sleepy. I had oatmeal, tea, bacon strips, one slice of French toast and grape juice for breakfast. I took a multi-vitamin, folic acid, Kytril, Fluconazale (an anti-fungal drug) and Acyclovir (anti-herpes). My blood counts were WBC 0.8, HCT 29.3 and PLT 71. White blood cells are what fights infection and my count was very low. I walked for twenty minutes and felt tired but sat in a chair for a while. The nurses liked me to get out of bed as much as possible as it was best for me.

While I was resting, Sandy Solomon telephoned and asked what specific things she could ask in prayer to help me. I said, "Pray that my blood counts grow to be normal, that I continue to live and thrive, and for a healthy body and immune system." Sandy attended 5:30 Mass at St. Pat's on Saturday and 10:30 Sunday services at First Presbyterian. Wow! I would be prayed up in

There But For the Grace of God

two churches by one woman! Sandy and I believed in the culture of life and supported President Bush. We didn't understand how some Catholics were not pro-life or how some were pro-life yet vote Democrat.

Gov. Pataki signed a bill to establish a cord blood center in Syracuse, according to Nurse Heidi. She was excited to share this news and said she would not have understood it if it hadn't been for me. I just hoped that it would happen soon but I have not seen it happen yet.

I took a shower while sitting in a chair. Also I had an IV for nausea and a Kytril pill. I was tired but still took an Ambien sleeping pill at 9 pm -- and at 2 AM I was wide awake again and opening mail. Bill hollered out in the night, "Help, help, help" so I woke him up. I was concerned the nurses would hear him and think something was wrong.

My blood counts were listed on a white board near my bedside each day. On November 4th, my WBC was 0.7, HCT (red) 29.2 and PLT (platelets) 51. I weighted 177. I received my cocktail of multi-vitamin, K, folic acid, Acyclovir and Fluconazale. Bill went to have breakfast in the cafeteria. I had bacon, French toast, oatmeal, cranberry juice and tea while I watched the news on TV. The lead story was that Saddam Hussein was found guilty and received a death sentence. I walked for twenty minutes and then Bill and I read the paper after which we dozed off. The doctors seemed to want me to eat as much as possible. My usual breakfast was a protein smoothie when I was not hospitalized.

Lunch choices were not to my liking so a nurse brought me some tomato soup. While Bill and I watched the Mass televised throughout the hospital, Mary Lou called. She had Bill meet her husband Al at the front of the hospital so Al could give Bill the laundry Mary Lou had done for me. I continued watching the Mass, and was surprised to see Bill on TV receiving communion, and after Mass talking to the priest. When Bill came back to my hospital room he brought communion to me. He was such a sweetheart to do that.

My supper was a hamburger and fruit cup, after which I showered. Each day I showered and it usually exhausted me. Tonight though, I was full of energy. My sister Sue had sent a tape on which she prayed the rosary, and I prayed along with her not once but twice. I offered up my prayers for the sanctification of embryonic life, the wisdom of voters, for pro-life issues and all those names on my prayer list as well as those who had no one to pray for them. As I read my Bible, I remembered all those Republican workers who telephoned me to campaign. When I told them about my cancer and the adult stem cell transplant, each said they would pray for me.

My letter on pro-life candidates had been published in the Tioga County *Courier* on November 1, which was also the date of my second adult stem cell transplant. Praise the Lord!

I had chicken noodle broth at 9:45 PM because I felt hollow and hungry.

At midnight I had a sleeping pill. I got the same medicines each day so I had stopped writing them down daily. Anything new I'd write down.

November 6th was my seventh day in the hospital but the fifth day since my transplant. My WBC was 0.3, HCT was 28.5 and my PLT was 36. Nurse Donna told me that this would be a busy day due to a new transplant patient being admitted. I volunteered to talk with either the patient or family as this was my second adult stem cell transplant and I might be of help with questions and fears.

My breakfast consisted of oatmeal, one slice of bacon and one slice French toast. After Bill has his cafeteria breakfast, he was going to look for a convenience store to buy me a softer toilet paper as the hospital toilet tissue was coarse and rough.

I stubbed my toe and it bled big time. I forgot my platelets were so low. I had to have the toe bandaged. Dr. Gentile told me I had multiple fractures in my pelvis from prior cancer and that was why my bones ache – as well as the normal arthritis that accompanies aging.

Bill returned from his walk with a newspaper and toilet paper. I did my hallway stroll and then we shared the newspaper. He watched TV and I said a rosary again with my sister's rosary tape. I napped for about twenty minutes until Mass at noon.

Nurse Holly informed me I had a visitor from long ago. It was one of my 1970s religion class students, Joan Meyers Delaney. That was a treat to see her again and I swear she hadn't aged a day. I received calls from friends and lots of mail which always lifted my spirits and made the time go faster.

I received my medicines from Nurse Donna who apologized for neglecting me (she didn't) due to the new patient who was pretty sick. I offered up prayers for other patients and our nurses, doctors, caregivers and families.

After supper I received my first shot of Neupogen in my left arm to help increase blood supply. Nurse Heidi was so smooth it barely hurt. She gave us paperwork on what to do after discharge. I finished the evening watching the Country Music Awards and heard so many inspiring songs of faith and life. It was a joy to listen to the show.

As I fell asleep, I remembered that the following day, November 7th, would have been my parents' 70th wedding anniversary. It was Pat and Dick Franz's 53rd anniversary. In a couple of weeks, Bill and I would celebrate 46 years of marriage. I offered up prayers for all of us.

Nurse Mike checked on me all night, which was considerate – except that I woke up every time, so I was exhausted in the morning. Krys called from Australia at 5:30 AM which also woke me. Bill started packing at 9 AM and

Mike and Bill talked for much of that time, so I feel like I was in a sleepy trance. After breakfast, Dr. Graziano gave me a check-up and medicines. My blood counts were WBC 0.2, HCT 26.4 and PLT 23.

Bill left for Owego so I turned off the phone, closed the blinds and went back to sleep for an hour. LuAnne cleaned my room and shower. When Nurse Robin made my bed the CODE button went off and nurses came running, thinking I coded (meaning, my heart stopped). That caused some excitement in my room!

The woman from Mineola called the wrong number again. We ended up talking about how over 400,000 people have been treated with adult stem cells, and I was able to stress that these therapies did not involve any embryonic tissue. God works in mysterious ways. This woman called for someone else and ended up talking with me twice now. Usually folks just say "I'm sorry" and hang up!

My sister Sue and her friend Mary called from Florida. Mary sent the Rochester article to her son in Michigan as his church had never mentioned adult stem cell and cord blood research. Mary thought cord blood might have helped her husband, who had unfortunately passed away by then. I received many phone calls while Nurse Della was fixing my chest wound and taking blood.

Tonight I felt cold, then warm, bowel pain then not, headache and ear discomfort then not. What was going on? The nurse gave me Oxycodine and I was able to sleep.

I was up at 6 AM due to a lot of loud noise at the nurses' desk. When Nurse Della came into my room later, I asked of there was a surprise party going on. She said no -- just employees coming on duty.

I took my usual litany of pills with breakfast, but threw them up in the toilet. Dr. Gentile and Laura, NP were there right after I threw up. I had a bag of platelets infused into me. I took my other medicines and could barely read my handwritten notes. Sandy and Sarah visited and brought me skin lotions but I kept falling asleep and wasn't very good company. My WBC was 0.1, ACT 24.7 and PLT 24.

Madeline, my spiritual advisor, prayed with me and patted my left hand. I cried over the election results as those like me needing adult stem cell research for their lives may be lost in the embryonic struggle and agenda of the majority of Democrats. I read my mail and then attempted to take a bath but I felt very shaky and clammy. I tried drinking some soup but dozed off with the bowl of soup in my hand. That got messy fast! I tried walking and said a rosary to keep me going but had to finish the rosary in bed.

The following day, I noticed that my handwriting was getting worse as my blood counts fell: WBC 0.4, HCT 25.1 and PLT 23. Nurse Traci gave me shots and medicines as I was eating breakfast. She wanted me up but I had to rest a while as I got very little sleep due to more noisy people at the desk that morning. I was in tears as I called Mary Lou and asked her for help. As there was generally no one around in the daytime, I tried to sleep. I walked briefly, rested, and then walked again. I threw up again at suppertime and briefly at x-ray. I developed a temperature of 101.2.

Mike McCormick, a friend from high school who now lived in Florida, called to tell me he was praying for me. I certainly needed prayer at just that time and God provided it. I was so out of it I couldn't do my daily Bible readings. I don't remember my conversations with Sarah and Sandy when they visited.

The next day my WBC was 0.1, HCT 21.8 and PLT 22. I had a chest x-ray taken. Dr. Gentile asked about my co-pay for Neupogen shots and I told her I had no insurance for prescriptions as I had exhausted my limit. They x-rayed my lungs as I had another fever. I received two bags of blood transfusions. I rested on and off all day. I did read cards but felt as limp as a strand of spaghetti.

Ten days after my transplant, it was hard to read my shaky handwriting but the blood counts were obvious. WBC 1.4, HCT is 27.3 and PLT were 25. I spent a lot of time walking, very slowly, sometimes with Bill and sometimes alone.

Jane called from Vegas and got me to laugh. She saw a show, *Bottoms Up*, featuring Gennifer Flowers, and there was a big red heart with Bill Clinton's picture in it. Gennifer said not to confuse her with Monica. I laughed and laughed as only in Vegas does stuff like that seems to happen. Laughter is such good medicine.

Nurse Marcia gave me my sixth Neupogen shot. I was also given Gentamicin to fight bacteria.

There was no mail as it was Veterans Day and the post office was closed, so that meant no cards. Craig called and we laughed and cried together. He had been ill and couldn't get to the hospital to be with me as he did last time.

On November 12, I woke up at 6 AM, so hot that I took off my pajamas. My WBC was 9.4, HCT was 29.9 and PLT was 35. I hoped that with these counts I would be able to go home, have no more Neuprogin shots, get some good sleep and get rid of a headache I'd been sporting for several days. I wanted Bill to shave my head as my hair was falling out in clumps. Dr. Gentile wanted me to use a Sitz-bath for a sore bottom. She said I could go home the next day if I had no fever. I called Jane in Palm Springs and Sarah called from Owego so I told them the latest on me.

Bill attended Mass as I watched on TV. The priest said America was blessed by God as we shared with those who had less food and resources than we do. The Nigerian village that he was from had no water to cook with or no sticks to make a cook fire. They waited for rain to get their water. The people celebrated praise for three or four hours in joy to the Lord. We have taken so much for granted in this country and I wondered if anyone really appreciated how fortunate they were to live in the United States.

Dr. Gentile was cutting me off fluids. The lab said my stool was infected with bacteria although the nurses found that hard to believe. The doctor was putting me on Flagyl which in the past had caused me to have headaches. When Nurse Donna told Bill that I was under quarantine and that Bill would have to wear a mask and gown, he turned white as a ghost and blew out of there so fast that the nurses laughed. I wished he had slowed down long enough to take a few things home, like my laundry. I was on all antibiotics now and finishing the last of the saline solution. The lab said my bowel issue was due to an organism called c-diff which is found in the intestines of healthy people. However, apparently in some people taking antibiotics, this germ can cause diarrhea, which is what happened with me. Just my luck!

On a lighter note, Tyler, my grandson, informed me he was shaving his head so he'd be bald like his granny.

I wrote a letter to the Syracuse newspaper entitled "Adult Stem Cell Transplants Done in Syracuse" after reading a letter to the editor that showed complete ignorance of the topic. I guess folks don't know that adult stem cell transplants can be done in Syracuse. I didn't know if they would print my letter, but as I never heard from them I guess they didn't.

November 13 was the twelfth day after my transplants, and my blood counts were WBC 22, HCT 30.4 and PTL 39. I weigh 176 pounds. At my midnight evaluation, Nurse Debbie woke me after only ten minutes of heavy sleep and I was like a zombie thereafter, catching twenty minutes of sleep here, ten minutes there. I tried listening to tapes of Priory monks chanting, MariJohn's singing, and Sue Ann praying the rosary, but nothing helped me relax.

I realized what had initiated the irritation in my peri-anal area was the spot where the measuring cups in the toilet join. The ridge was just where the soreness in my nether region was! I will be so glad not to have my bowel movements and urine measured constantly.

In the morning, I received another bag of potassium by infusion and discharge instructions from Laura, NP and Nurse Donna. And they told me I was going home today! Hoorah!

Prior to leaving I received another shot of Neupogen which Nurse Heidi described as Miracle Grow for white blood cells.

Bill and I drove straight home from Syracuse. Bill dropped my many prescriptions off at the drugstore while I stayed home eating soup. I needed my walker as I was very unstable. Becky from Home Health Care taught Bill how to clean my port and left us supplies. I was soooo tired and had chills, but we had an hour of paperwork to do with HHC and then I slept for a couple of hours.

On November 14, my first full day home, Bill and I discussed where to go for my blood work and I won. We drove to Lourdes Hospital in Binghamton. I lacked a billing code on my blood work order so I called Dusty at Dr. Cooke's office to get the insurance code. There was no one at Lourdes who knew how to use a "port" so they took blood the old fashioned way -- from my arm -- and faxed the results to the Syracuse transplant unit. On our way home we picked up sandwiches. It took me two days to eat one sandwich. I rested most of the day except for talking to family via telephone. Bill went out for supper.

My second full day home, I took a shower using Press & Seal over my port to keep the bandages dry. After getting dressed, I stood in the driveway while Bill shaved my head. We walked to the corner and back. Ed Mitch hugged me and visited with us but I became so tired that we went home. I had a bowl of tomato soup for lunch and took a nap. I ate the rest of the soup for supper and read computer messages. I slept badly all night as I was either very cold or too warm.

The third full day home I felt so cold and tired. Sarah came to stay with me while Bill met his coffee group at the Parkview. I listened to phone messages, one of which was from a United Healthcare nurse. Broome and Tioga County (where I live) were in a state of emergency due to flooding.

We got up at 6 AM to be at the Syracuse Hospital by 8 AM. It wasn't easy with so many roads flooded but we found a way to get there. I had my port removed with no needles to numb the area as it was less painful that way. The doctor literally just yanked it out. I next met with Dr. Gentile about the results of my blood work done in the lab. Some of my blood counts were good -- WBC 8.8, HCT 39 -- but my PLT was still low. The doctor recommended that if I traveled, I should stay away from Texas and Florida due to fungus. Nevada would be all right because it was dry. I still had loose bowels due to the c-diff germ.

When we arrived back in Owego I napped and then we went grocery shopping and walked. Bill went out for supper but I stayed in and had a breakfast shake for supper. I made phone calls, read computer messages and wrote the Syracuse *Post Standard* about adult stem cell research. Sue Ballard called and wanted me to get my book finished.

I was awake from 1 to 2 AM, but then fell asleep. I got up around 9 AM and had Boost for breakfast as well as all my pills. I still had the "trots" and chills and rested in my nightgown and robe all day. Dan Mieczkowski stopped to visit and brought food for Thanksgiving dinner, courtesy of his parents who live on our street. He said they prayed for me during grace.

I called Brenda, who said I gave her gumption. If I could go through what I was going through, then she could strive to do more even though she has MS.

Again I had Boost for breakfast and I took over an hour getting all my pills down.

I made up a packet on adult stem cell research for paraplegics to give a young man we'd met at the drugstore. His dad fell off a roof and was in a wheelchair.

It was 23 degrees when we left again for Syracuse. I weighed in at 172 in clothes and shoes. The doctor said my chest was good and that my red blood cells were in normal range, with my white count and platelets almost normal. My temperature was 97.1 which was normal for me. I could stop taking Flagyl. Hoorah! I still felt cold from inside my body to outside, which I thought was weird.

We stopped at a mall where I did a little walking, as Dr. Gentile says I needed to walk to build my strength. I called Craig and told him Dr. Gentile said I was healthy enough to come for Christmas as long as the children were not sick

I was so thankful to be alive to celebrate Thanksgiving Day. I watched Bill attempt to clean the turkey by using the water spray attachment on the kitchen sink and tried not to laugh. I helped by telling him each step to clean the turkey so he didn't have to read the instructions. As dinner cooked, we watched some of Macy's Parade but the commentators talked over the band music so we gave up, had dinner and took a nap. I called Brenda and thanked her for the sweatshirt she sent me from Colorado that said, "Her Ladyship." I love anything to do with England. All our children and many friends called.

Thanksgiving was such an exhausting day I was still tired the next morning. At 5:30 AM, Bill fell partway down the second story stairs but was okay. It scared us both.

We walked up and down the street and then took naps. I started Flagyl again because of loose bowels, but then stopped after 24 hours because my stomach was bothering me. My bones ached which was probably due to the humidity and lousy weather.

I received a card in the mail for a year of masses from a stranger named Jo S., of Port Leyden, New York. She wrote, "May God who sends the choicest gifts of flowers, sun and dew, now add the very precious one of perfect health for you. Thank you for sharing your story with us in the *North Country Catholic*. You are playing a big part in educating the public in stem cell transplants using adult stem cells, rather than the sinful practice of embryonic. Every baby saved will be praying for you, I'm sure. Sincerely, Jo S."

Nov. 26 was our 46th wedding anniversary. Bill attended Mass while I watched Mass on TV. I would have loved to have attended Mass in person, but there would have been too many parishioners coughing and sneezing, and my system couldn't handle that yet.

Bill and I took our walk and then put up our Christmas tree. I was so cold that I wrapped up in blankets even though it was 50 degrees outside. My neighbor Rachel knitted me four caps, using all different stitching, to cover my bald head and keep my body heat in my body.

Our children and grandchildren called to wish us Happy Anniversary.

On Monday, I received good news from Laura in Syracuse. She said I could stop taking potassium and magnesium tablets and start taking Bactrim. I would have loved to be taking nothing at all; I was so tired of taking pills.

Bill and I walked on the street today. Ed Mitch gave me a hug, a decorative sled for the front porch, stationery and mini-pies. What a treat when I was just out for a walk!

Craig drove south from Malone and Bill and I drove north from Owego, and we all met at Syracuse University Hospital Regional Oncology Center. Craig went to my appointment with Dr. Gentile and Nurse Kathy. My platelet count had dropped so I was taken off Bactrim. I had lost two pounds. The doctor said I had aching bowels due to the chemo that was still in my body and that I should eat a bland diet. She added that I could make an appointment with Dr. Sheth at Broome Oncology for Zometa and blood work per her instructions. After the two hour car ride back home we arrived just in time for Nurse Kathy's phone call; she said that due to my work-up results, I needed to be taking in more fluids.

The last day of November, I gave up naps and using a walker. I walked on the street all by myself. Praise the Lord!

Sarah drove me to my appointment with Dr. Sheth at Broome Oncology. I had blood work done that showed WBC 3.6, HCT 35.8, platelets 90 and HGB 11.9. I received an infusion of Zometa to help strengthen my bones. As I lacked enough fluid in my body, it was difficult for the nurse to find a good vein to insert the needle for the Zometa.

I woke up in the night feeling nauseous, achy, and covered in sweat. I had to wash myself and change my pajamas. This was from the Zometa infusion. I felt weak for the next couple of days. I called Laura, RNP in Syracuse and she said she thought my hormones played a part of the problem.

The Binghamton *Press & Sun-Bulletin* called asking permission to print a letter on adult stem cell therapies that I had e-mailed them. Even though I was going through cancer treatments again, I did not let it stop me from educating people on adult stem cells.

I did my Bible readings, watched EWTN and rested in the Lord in the quiet of my bedroom. Colossians 3:24 says: "Whatever your work is, put your heart into it as if it were for the Lord and not for men, knowing that the Lord will repay you by making you his heirs. It is Christ the Lord that you are serving." I had another big day for me as I drove the car by myself. This was the first time since my latest transplant. I walked alone outdoors for over thirty minutes where I saw a neighbor, Dave Evans, who told me to keep writing letters on adult stem cell treatments.

I saw a fantastic TV show called "Animals in the Womb" put on by National Geographic. How I wished people cared about humans in the womb as much as they did animals. This program showed what a miracle life was and I didn't understand how anyone could watch a show like this and still be in favor of aborting and killing innocent lives.

WOW! I received a Christmas card from Vice President and Mrs. Cheney and also one from President and Laura Bush, plus several Christmas cards from English and European friends. They perked me up as I read them over and over.

I had to renew some prescriptions which cost almost $400. I weaned myself off Protonix, which was an expensive pill, as I didn't seem to have to acid reflux anymore now that I was not taking so many strong medicines. I could hardly wait until 2007 rolled around and my prescription coverage starts again. I walked every day unless the weather was icy as I needed to regain my strength.

Every day as I walked down the street, I said a rosary and prayers for people. For meals I heated up some of Fran Kobziewicz's dishes of food she made that were stored in our freezer.

A month later, I made my last trip to see Dr. Gentile in Syracuse as she said I was doing fine and I could return to Broome Oncology for check-ups every three months. We agreed on no Zometa or Thalomid for me because of side effects. I started taking vitamins again, especially calcium for my bones. When I asked about traveling she said there was no problem, as long as I was traveling by car.

I responded to a mistaken comment on embryonic stem cell research that was printed in the Reader's Column of the Owego *Pennysaver*. I also wrote to Art as well as the stranger friend, Jo S. who had the year's worth of masses said for me. I attended a Charismatic Healing Mass where Fr. Boniface prayed over me and I went to the floor resting in the Holy Spirit. Fr. Boniface told me whenever he saw me he saw great faith in me and assured me that God would use me in many ways.

On December 21, 2006 -- the first day of winter -- and I was feeling fit enough to enroll in Curves Exercise Program again. Sue, Gail and Candy had a decorated table-top Christmas tree for me and also gave me a basket of goodies. There was a card signed by many women who worked out when I did prior to my transplant stay in the hospital. I had tears in my eyes and thanked them. I wore surgical gloves to work out in order to prevent bacteria from any machine getting on my hands as I exercised. Even so, I felt so "normal." I walked while praying a rosary and as I read the National Right to Life newspaper.

Craig called to say everyone in his house was healthy, so Bill and I packed up and headed to Malone, New York for Christmas with Craig, Julie, Abbey and Olivia. Again I felt so "normal." I would have *looked* it if my hair had grown back in. Their home was decorated beautifully for Christmas and we had carolers our first night there. Christmas Eve everyone went to church but me, as I still didn't expose myself to crowds. After Mass they picked me up for a Christmas Eve meal at Julie's parents' home. The following morning, we watched the girls open their gifts from Santa and family, and that was the first time we'd done that. Later on we had a brunch, but Abbey vomited and had a temperature of 101. Julie took her to the hospital where she was diagnosed with strep throat. Bill and I left for home the next day, Boxing Day, as now Julie was also ill with strep throat and I couldn't be exposed any more than I already had been.

My scripture meditation was "Be assured that as you continue to witness, pray, share the gospel, and serve, the Holy Spirit will be working. And when you get to heaven, you may be amazed at how many people are there in part because of your life. How grateful they will be! And how grateful will you be that God chose to use you so powerfully."[7] Two days after Christmas, I had an appointment with Mary Benz, NP, because I was feeling weak, coughing and my throat was sore. She put me on a Z Pac of pills. I was soooo tired but still did some laundry, read e-mails and said two rosaries.

I had blood work done at Broome Oncology which showed a WBC of 4.10, an HGB of 11.1, an HCT of 32.6 and a PLT of 60.5. Dr. Sheth was happy and gave me paperwork for a 100-day check-up.

I received a letter from Jane Doty which meant a lot to me. It said, "You are a special person -- not only to me but to God. I thank Him so much for all the things He has brought to me through you. May the Lord's healing grace be with you always. We go back to 1958. God was so good to me by all the people He had brought into my life. You are one of them. I love you -- Janie."

Another special friend wrote, "This card is for a very special lady whom I'm privileged to call my friend. Hope you had a wonderful time celebrating Christmas time with family and friends. I will be thinking of you and I also wish you health and happiness in the New Year. Christmas brings many gifts but none more precious than the gift of your friendship. Love, Krys."

Lastly Marge Stanton wrote, "Dear Carol and Bill, Hope things are going well and that you, Carol, are healing well. Looking for that miracle that we know God can do. God Bless you both. You are in my thoughts and prayers. We serve an awesome God."

I met Gloria Felice and she remarked to me, "How wonderful that you know what mission God wants you to do with your life."

Chapter 30: Mission Year 2007

New Year's Day was spent quietly and with friends who stopped by to check on me. The first Thursday of the month, I attended a Leukemia, Lymphoma and Myeloma Support Group meeting -- and I drove myself! I couldn't get over the fact that I drove and didn't need caregivers! I wore my tee-shirt that said, "Former Embryo." I learned from the lecture that drinking plenty of fluids, eating protein, taking Vitamin B and exercising would combat fatigue. Later at home, my foot and leg fell asleep while I was on the phone and when I tried to stand and walk I fell, skinning my arm and landing with such a thud that Bill rushed into the room. I bandaged my arm and would check for bruises later.

Oh boy, did I ever ache for days from my fall.

I found in my Bible a letter from a Florida Southern College student dated February 1984. She was working on a ride at Busch Gardens and I was in line wearing a button that said, "I am pro-life." The letter read: "Dear Carol, I had prayed for a while that the Lord would reveal someone to help me with my desire to help in the anti-abortion work. I never dreamed He'd answer my prayers at Busch Gardens and with someone who lives so far away. He is miraculous, isn't He? I just want to thank you for all your help. I want you to know that I was over-whelmed with all the literature you sent to me. I just hope I can do my part and be a good pro-life supporter. Please keep my ministry in your prayers. I want to get more people aware, and God-willing I will. To be honest, I didn't know if I'd hear from you. You must have thought it strange to be approached so abruptly in such a strange place. I just want to thank you for your quick response. I'll keep your work in my prayers. Thank you again for your help! God has used you in a dynamic way! Who knows? Maybe we will meet again if I ever get to New York! Take Care! Your friend, Susan C. P.S. I loved the healing story you sent. What a beautiful miracle. PTL."

Anne LeBlanc of Rochester Right to Life asked if I'd be willing to take part in a TV commentary with members and a doctor on stem cell research. It would probably be held on January 17, 2007. I said I'd be there if the snowstorms allowed me to get through!

Our buddy, George Hall, called to ask about the latest news on "Amniotic

Stem Cells Show Amazing Promise" that he read in the *Press*. Several other people called or e-mailed to make sure I knew of the article. My rag-tag army was ever vigilant in keeping me informed.

I received an e-mail from Cancer Advocacy Now and was so annoyed by their promotion of the embryonic stem cell bill in Congress that I wrote a scathing e-mail and requested my name be dropped from their mailings. Adult stem cell research has helped cancer patients, so they should be promoting adult stem cell research!

I picked up my last vial of Valtrex which prevented shingles and I saved $166 by having insurance. How wonderful and relaxing to know I had prescription insurance again.

Doris Camp, VFW Auxiliary, asked I would give a presentation in the spring on adult stem cell research and therapies. It would be open to the public and I agreed to do it.

I was so bummed over the embryonic stem cell vote in the House that I wore my "Former Embryo" shirt to Curves and kept wearing it all day, even to the dentist's office. Ronnie, an assistant to the dentist, was shocked to hear abortions were available in the ninth months of pregnancy. I gave her my testimony paper and a copy of the National Right to Life newspaper. I put ninety-five copies of the newspaper in four Catholic churches in my parish. I took one to the public library and handed out copies to close friends.

The Word Among Us meditation spoke directly to my heart and mind. "Brothers and sisters, Jesus is pouring so much into you because he sees the state of the world. Yes, he wants to make you happy; but he also wants to send you into a world of sadness, pain and division."[8] Lord, give me the strength to be your light to the world as I want to serve you.

I was energized by the following letter. "Dear Carol, I can not tell you what a joy it was to open up the mail we received from you today! How wonderful that your treatment has been successful and that you are spreading the word about the hope of adult stem cell transplants! Our organization is dedicated to pro-woman/pro-life solutions. I am sure you know our new governor is chomping at the bit regarding embryonic stem cell research and its future in New York. We are very happy to receive your membership. In April we would be traveling to Albany to meet legislators. Our visit usually centers on two issues and we meet in pairs throughout the day for scheduled visits with our state's lawmakers. We would be delighted to have you with us. We look forward to hearing from you. Feminists Choosing Life."

I was invited to participate in a twice-monthly half-hour TV program, "The Terri West Show," on a local access channel in Rochester. Bill and I drove through snow to get there, but it was worth it; Terri, the interviewer, found all the information was so interesting that she taped two shows. My

There But For the Grace of God

"before and after" photos were shown on the first taping. A banner of adult stem cell human therapies was hanging during the second taping. According to the technician taping the show, the format was a sort of pro-life version of The View, featuring Anne, Dr. Barb, Wilda, Carol, and me.

Next, Bill and I were on the road to Texas, Arizona and Nevada, dodging ice storms and snow in the eastern states. Every time we saw members of the military, we thanked them for their service. At the Tennessee Visitor Center, Bill and I shared information about adult stem cell transplant with the guide. I gave her the www.stemcellresearch.org site. When we ate lunch at Subway, we shared adult stem cell information with the clerks as we four were the only ones in the building. When we got to Dan's in Texas, we checked our e-mails. I received a note from Anne LaBlanc congratulating me on the good job I'd done during the interviews on the Terri West Show. Terri received lots of phone calls and the TV station director was considering producing DVDs of the two half-hour shows. Anne said to pat myself on the back. The episodes on which we appeared were a big hit with many callers. The show received the most calls of any of her programs.

At Mass on Sunday, Keith of the Knights of Columbus asked about my lime green Adult Stem Cell Transplant Survivor shirt. At the HEB grocery store two more men asked about my being an adult stem cell survivor. At the HEB checkout counter, an elderly lady asked me to watch her cart for her. When she returned, we spoke about adult stem cells. She blamed President Bush so I set her straight. She called her daughter, a Kansas resident, over to listen. The daughter took my card and said she'd go onto www.stemcellresearch.org, as well as Google my name. She asked if a sick friend could contact me and I said yes. I believe nothing is by chance and that my suffering is to help others.

I read the Austin *Statesman* and e-mailed them in reply to their editorial pushing embryonic research. I received an e-mail from the paper asking for confirmation of my letter and asking if my e-mail address can be published. I replied yes.

On a lighter note, I had to stitch up McBain the dog's favorite chew toy -- his Hillary Clinton doll!

I telephoned Brenda and told her how a tee-shirt design had come to my mind. So many people commented on my shirt that promoted adult stem cells saving lives; would they like to wear a version of their own? I asked her what she thought. I also told Terry when she called, and she said, "Do It!" I decided on "Adult stem cells saved my friend's life" as the slogan. I planned to sell them at cost or in some cases, give them away. I didn't want to make a profit on the shirts, but I'd prefer not to lose money on them, either. I tucked that idea away in my brain for another day.

February 8, 2007 was the 100th day since my latest adult stem cell transplant. We were in Las Vegas, Nevada. At a Honda dealership, a fellow mentioned my shirt and said, "Bush is an a--." I told the guy he didn't have correct information, and I explained about Congress voting down funding ethical embryonic and adult stem cell research and the circumstances of Bush's veto. I mentioned Senators Reid, Clinton and Schumer and the many Democrats who were not helping people like me to survive. Next we went to Red Rock Casino for lunch. A man behind the Players Club Desk asked about the saying on my sweatshirt. When I explained, he asked me to talk to another clerk whose dad had leukemia and no immune system. I gave them my card and the www.stemcellresearch.org site. Then I met Andy, who was sitting at a slot machine next to Bill. When I explained to Andy what my shirt meant, he had me pick his bonus on the machine because I was a living miracle. (He won a great deal of money.)

Another day, we drove with the Clears to Bonnie Springs Old Mining Town. In one shop the owner read my button and told me he was a cancer survivor, too. He asked about my treatment and I gave him a card and newspaper article. Back at our hotel, Terrible's, an employee using a walker commented on my shirt. I explained ASCT to her and she turned to a man and said, "Did you hear that?" He made a negative comment and blamed President Bush for vetoing stem cell research. I remarked, "You don't know what you are talking about." I then proceeded to set him straight on the facts of the matter. Bill said, "You chewed the guy a new a--hole." I thought I was calm but stern when I spoke to him! I guess there's a difference in how men and women answer -- or maybe I was tired of dealing with ignorance to the left and right of me!

I met with Dr. Clark Jean at the Comprehensive Cancer Center of Nevada for blood work and exam. My WBC was 3.6, red was slightly below normal and platelets were 80. He told me once a year Zometa would be all that was necessary as my bones were strong. I weighed in at 169 so he told me to lose some weight by walking. He was impressed with my looks. The IgA type of multiple myeloma that I had was not the worst of the strain; there are two varieties that are worse, and with IgM there was little to no help. I loved the fact that I didn't ache in my bones while in Nevada. Praise God for the dry desert climate.

We were on our way back east when we passed through Kingman, Arizona and had lunch at In-n-Out Burger. There a woman congratulated me on my adult stem cell transplant. Her friend, another multiple myeloma patient, was three years in remission after having an adult stem cell transplant. Her father-in-law was having an adult stem cell transplant as we spoke. What a small world!

There But For the Grace of God

When Bill and I attended Mass at St. Margaret Mary Catholic Church in Cedar Park, Texas, I wore the badge pin that Emy printed for me. As Bill used Purel to wash his hand after sharing the sign of Peace, he explained to the woman sitting next to him about me. A couple from Corpus Christi, TX talked to us after Mass. My bald head caught their attention, as she too was a cancer survivor but was battling two types of cancer. Her doctor had told her there were no stem cell successes with cancer, so she came to Austin to see other doctors. I told her that her Corpus Christi doctor must have been talking about embryonic stem cells, which had, so far, never helped any cancer patient. I gave her my card and I also gave my card to the Deacon and to the youth director as I left the church. Another man I encountered thought umbilical cords contained embryonic stem cells until I straightened him out. After church we stopped at the HEB Food Store where a clerk took off her cap to show me her hair loss from having chemo for breast cancer. We hugged and shared our stories.

Back at Daniel's house where I walked in the neighborhood, I stopped to chat with a young couple who had a child in a stroller. I asked if Texas collected umbilical cords. They only knew about private, individual collecting, so I explained about adult stem cells in cord blood and other information. I had the inclination to stop and speak to a woman weeding her shrubbery. I told her I envy her working with earth and explained why I could not. It seems she was a cervical cancer survivor. She said I was so brave to do an adult stem cell transplant. I have never thought of bravery, but thought I was intelligent to do it! When I got back to the house, I had a sore throat, runny nose, sneezing -- all allergy symptoms. My body wanted the Nevada climate, not Texas where allergens roam twelve months of the year! At the Post Office in Cedar Park, a woman standing in line behind me said she had an adult stem cell transplant done in Houston, Texas in April 2006 for leukemia. She said to keep wearing my shirts.

I sent a letter to Texas Gov. Rick Perry as well as a copy of the 72 adult stem cell therapies versus zero embryonic stem cell therapies from www.stemcellresearch.org, a copy of Dennis Turner's Parkinson adult stem cell transplant information, and of Laura D's spinal cord treatment with adult stem cells. I sent the same to Lance Armstrong as well as a tape of my story.

Terry phoned and told me, "Mom, I have seen a lot of very sick people with cancer at the hospital and you are blessed to be alive and doing so well. You look so good and I am so glad I have you as my mom." I give all the credit to the Great Physician and to those caring adult stem cell oncologists and doctors here on earth.

I wrote to the Austin *Statesman* about a misleading headline on stem cell research put out by the AP. Kathy Bergman called me from Owego, New York

Carol J. Franz

as she had seen the same article and was annoyed also.

I was contacted by Gene Tarne of Do No Harm and www.stemcellresearch.org on submitting my story to their site. Also in March, in Washington DC, there would be a briefing of members and staff of politicians, a press conference, and a wine reception by BOGOwines.com on the Hill. I was asked to share my story. All this would be taped so the video could be accessed via the internet site. Gene explained to me how fetal stem cells were being transplanted into human patients with disastrous results. An embryonic transplant killed a man, so mostly fetal stem cells are used.

Next I saw Dr. Dee Butler at the Austin Regional Clinic, who said that it wasn't allergies causing my coughing, wheezing and runny nose – it was an infection. He tested my lungs and determined I lacked oxygen, so he put me on puffers. He said I had reactive airway disease and prescribed a Z Pac as well as two inhalers, one of which was a steroid.

We started traveling back East and as we stopped at Bristol, Tennessee rest stop, Joyce and Jeffrey, two employees at the welcome center, asked me about my adult stem cell shirt. Bill and I explained how the Lord had blessed me. When we stopped at McDonald's for Bill's coffee, a couple asked us the difference between embryonic and adult stem cells. So many people inquired and I felt blessed that my Lord would use me in this way. If I didn't wear the shirts or badges a great number of people would still be uninformed.

Once we arrived back home in Owego, I ordered shirts from Susquehanna Printers that said, "Adult stem cells saved my Mom's life," "Adult stem cells saved my friend's life," "Adult stem cells saved my sister's life" and a shirt for me that said, "Survivor, adult stem cell transplant, NOT embryonic." I ordered several of the "friend" shirts and gave them to my friends at cost -- or if they couldn't afford it, just gave it to them, period. I got my first request on line for "shirts" from Mary Kay in Owego and Mary Hinchcliffe in California. Mary from California was one of the first to notice something was wrong with me at the class reunion.

When Bill and I had breakfast at the American Legion, Ralph asked me which party supported adult stem cell research. I told him NOT Clinton, Schumer nor Hinchey's party, as they wouldn't even listen to me. I let him draw his own conclusion.

Whenever charitable or political groups call me for a donation, I explained how my money was going for my mission of spreading the word of adult stem cell research and therapies. People seemed genuinely interested to learn the facts of ASCR and many said they would pray for me.

Sarah Hall joined me at a social for the Leukemia, Lymphoma and Myeloma Society held in Endicott, New York. I wore one of my shirts, and a cancer survivor thought my shirt represented embryonic stem cell research.

She didn't know a thing about adult stem cell research. If cancer patients didn't know the truth, why did I expect healthy people to? I had spent the last five years of my life learning about this – but then, as my dad would say, "my elevator goes all the way to the top."

Bill and I met Fr. Boniface for lunch at the Cellar Restaurant. Father shared stories he told in Africa about me and my positive attitude through the adversity I have experienced. He told Bill I was doing God's calling. It was not Carol's work but God's work, he said, and I was gifted. This helped Bill understand that all the speaking and traveling I did concerning adult stem cell therapies and research was a God-given mission.

I received inquiries about adult stem cell treatments from several people in Texas, New York and Pennsylvania as well as from the *Pennysaver* in Owego and Channel 34-TV in Binghamton. My spiritual reading had said things would start happening rapidly and I could see it in my adult stem cell mission. I received touching letters like this: "Thank you for writing your letter regarding stem cells. There is so much misinformation floating around. I have an adult son with a spinal cord injury and [I am] researching facilities and physicians who are doing adult stem cell implants. Would you mind sharing where you were treated and any information you have? Many thanks and may you continue to live in health and prosperity."

Suzie Wolcott called to inform me that Rev. Dr. Tadeusz Pacholczyk, Director of Education at the National Catholic Bioethics Center was speaking at the Guthrie Clinic, so I quickly got ready and drove to Sayre, Pennsylvania to hear him. After a loud doctor who appeared to be anti-religion stood up and spouted off to Fr. Tad, I raised my hand and Fr. Tad called on me. I told of my being alive due to two adult stem cell transplants and that I had a new immune system and blood supply. When I sat down I remarked to the doctor sitting next to me that if the loudmouth doctor had his way, I'd be dead. The doctor next to me just grinned at me. I really had to get ready for my trip to Washington, DC, but I was glad I took the time to make the thirty-minute trip to the Guthrie Clinic.

Chapter 31: Mrs. Franz Goes to Washington, DC

It was snowing as we left Owego for Washington, DC. We got there around 3:00 PM and toured the WWII Memorial. Bill keyed up his dad, Richard, on a database and it showed Franz soldiers with first names from A to W. I took lots of pictures as I walked around in my lime-green, long-sleeved "Survivor, adult stem cell transplant, NOT embryonic" tee-shirt. We walked by the White House and past several impressive buildings that looked like the government buildings we saw in England when we lived there. We checked into our room on the eleventh floor. The young man was taken with my story and gave us concierge privileges during our stay. I was scheduled to meet the other presenters at the Family Research Council at 10:30 AM Monday. This was my first experience in talking about adult stem cell research on Capital Hill and I was eager.

On Monday morning at breakfast, two gentlemen read my shirt and stopped to talk to me. It seemed they too would be on Capital Hill with Do No Harm. One was Dr. Zannos Grekos, a cardiologist from Bonita Springs, Florida, and Douglas T. Rice, an adult stem cell recipient for congestive heart failure from the states of Washington and Texas. Prior to arriving at the Family Research Council, Bill and I made a visit to St. Patrick's Church and prayed. We took cabs from the FRC to the Dirksen Senate Office Building and the Russell Building with an Assistant FRC Director, who guided us to the offices where we had appointments. Bill, two other adult stem cell survivors and I had meetings all day Monday and Tuesday with either Senators or their staff. We were accompanied by Dr. David Prentice of the Family Research Council; Colin McGuckin, a professor of regenerative medicine at the School of Clinical and Laboratory Sciences/ Haematological Sciences, University of Newcastle upon Tyne (UK); and Richard Doerflinger, Deputy Director of the US Conference of Catholic Bishops, as well as various members of their staffs.

The two other speakers besides me were men. Steven Sprague had a cord blood transplant more than ten years ago for leukemia. There was no bone marrow match for him but a woman had donated her daughter's cord blood, so a stranger's blood saved Stephen's life. Doug suffered from congestive heart failure and diabetes. He was told he had only a couple months to live. An adult stem cell transplant from himself to himself saved his life. The technique was the work of doctors in Pittsburgh but the FDA had not approved the procedure in the USA so patients as well as doctors had to go out of the country. Doug went to Bangkok, Thailand to have the procedure done. They drew his blood, sent his blood to Israel where the adult stem cells needed to help his heart were pulled from the blood and sent back to Bangkok. It was a forty-five minute procedure to replace the blood back into his body through a catheter. It regenerated his heart. Blood flow increased from 11% to 30% and within weeks he was feeling normal again. Some of the adult stem cells stayed in his heart but 50% also went looking for other problems and improved his kidneys and pancreas. He still had heart disease and diabetes when I met him, but no longer needed to take so much insulin.

Can you imagine being that sick and having to fly twenty hours because the Food and Drug Administration was processing adult stem cell procedures the same way they do new pills or drugs on the market? Most adult stem cells are taken from your own body or relatives so there was very little chance your body would reject them and they do not cause tumors or make you sicker. While the FDA fiddles around, over 750,000 people die yearly in the USA from heart disease while many might benefit from this procedure. I am glad the FDA tests drugs a long time, but adult stem cells are natural, not a drug. Oh, maybe that's why. Natural, not a profit-making drug! The FDA has approved a morning after abortion pill from which women have had terrible consequences, but they have not approved using your own adult stem cells to save your life from many different diseases and injuries. What's the logic in that thinking?

Several influential senators weren't there personally, but had sent staff members to hear our testimonies. These senators included John Isakson from Georgia, Claire McCaskell from Missouri, Saxby Chambliss from Georgia, Elizabeth Dole from North Carolina, and Mitch McConnell from Kentucky. We personally told our stories to Senators Norm Coleman of Minnesota, Chuck Grassley of Iowa, Dr. Tom Coburn of Oklahoma, Bob Corker of Tennessee, Jim Bunning of Kentucky and Sam Brownback of Kansas. Senator Corker, TN passed by me in a hallway, stopped and said, "I believe in what your shirt says." Senator Grassley had another group waiting to speak to him, but once he heard our stories he stayed longer as he wanted to know more. Everyone we spoke to had that reaction.

Well, almost everyone. As the men passed New York Senator Chuck Schumer in the hallway, they all stopped. I was lagging behind the men and as I arrived they were chatting away about nothing. I told Schumer I was alive due to adult stem cell research and asked him to vote for funding the type of research that had saved my life instead of the Stem Cell Act S5 that only funded embryonic research. I told him over 400,000 humans had been treated with adult stem cells.

He informed me that doctors and scientists told him thousands of humans had been treated and helped with embryonic stem cells.

I replied, "That's not true."

I guess you don't tell a Senator that something isn't true because he got huffy. He said, "I am for both. Are you for both?"

I replied, "I support adult and ethical stem cell research."

He said with a sneer, "Ethical," then looked at my shirt, which said, "Survivor adult stem cell transplant, not embryonic" and said, "It's your religion."

I said, "Religion has no part in it. It's science." I added, "I don't believe in cloning."

He replied, "I don't either."

I wanted to ask where he thought he was going to get enough embryos without cloning, but I just walked away saying, "Thank you for not representing me."

He sputtered and hollered, "I represent a lot of people, not just you. 77% of New Yorkers support embryonic stem cell research."

I knew that was questionable as polls never ask you what type of stem cell research you support; they just ask whether you support stem cell research. Most New Yorkers are clueless that there are different kinds.

As I walked away he was still hollering and sputtering. I thought, "What a Kodak Moment. Where are the TV cameras when you want them?"

I was lectured by Bill and Doug for even attempting to talk to my Senator.

We also spoke at the Heritage Foundation, a renowned conservative think tank and bastion of traditional American values. We attended a wine reception in the Dirksen Senate Office Building arranged by BOGOwines.com. Illinois-based BOGO donated money from each sale of their fine Italian wines to adult stem cell research, and each bottle stated that fact. It was sold on-line. It used to be sold in liquor stores at one time but people pushing for embryonic research raised a fuss and the stores asked BOGO to remove the wines. This wasn't a contest in stem cell research. Science has shown adult stem cell research regenerates life. We survivors again told our stories and we were taped for TV, radio and You Tube. Lots of Senate staffers showed up for the free food and wines. Gee, what a surprise!

President Bush sent a congratulatory letter to the Do No Harm Coalition, www.stemcellresearch.org. The letter was very uplifting as the First Family thanked everyone for their efforts. Due to the media's confusion over the issue, so many people thought that President Bush was against stem cell research, which was not true. He was in favor of adult and ethical embryonic stem cell research, and his administration was the only one to ever fund both. Eventually pictures of the survivors and the wine reception were posted at www.bogowines.com.

Doug and I were interviewed for the radio at the Family Research Council. Dr. Prentice encouraged me to keep wearing my shirts and spreading the word that way.

Bill, Doug, Richard and I traveled to Annapolis, Maryland to speak at a Senate Legislative Committee meeting. We met up with Dr. Roselle Abraham, a John Hopkins University Cardiologist; Yuval Levin, a fellow in Ethics and Public Policy; and Wendy Wright, President of Concerned Women of America as well as three women who work for the Conference of Catholic Bishops. In Maryland, there was equal funding for both adult and embryonic stem cell research. A bill was being considered that would give priority funding for embryonic research. The irony was that requests for grants to fund adult stem cell research were more common in Maryland than requests to fund embryonic research because adult research was so successful. Why would you want to work on a loser?

Anyway, the Bill SB 59 Stem Cell Enhancement Act of 2007 by Senator Lenett was withdrawn for review as we survivors, doctors and advocates told our stories and gave our speeches. Our group was elated and Richard said it was due to the survivors being there. Another bill, Retrieval of Oocytes-Prohibition (eggs from women) was discussed, both pro and con. Pro-life and Pro-choice women were united in fighting against using women as egg donors for embryonic research. Newspapers on university campus were advertising from $500 to $6,000 for egg donors. Some young women have died and many more have suffered infertility, pain, or infection due to the procedure. These young women may have not realized they would be jeopardizing their future as mothers.

Bill and I walked the adorable narrow streets of Annapolis before driving home to Owego. I sent out an e-mail of my trip and received many responses, but my favorite was from Ann in Rochester, New York, who wrote, "As I sit here, all I can think is how proud I am of what you have done, if that makes sense. I'm proud to know you. It just tickles me pink that you have been such a witness to the truth, that you thought of the idea of that sweatshirt and that you probably put Senator Schumer in a kind of uncomfortable spot. Hooray."

At home, Bill and I had breakfast at the Owego Treadway where the hostess told me she loved my haircut. I got that a lot as my hair was really short but starting to grow back. Bill told her it was from chemo. She answered that she too had chemo. I told her my adult stem cell transplant story and gave her a copy of the Do No Harm listings of therapies. She shared it with a waitress whose boyfriend had leukemia.

Within the next few days, I was interviewed in our living room by Steve Craig of Channel 34 News, the Binghamton ABC affiliate. I thought it went rather well considering it was the media, and the lime green shirt really showed up. I was surprised to see that a photo of Doug Rice (who had received an adult stem cell transplant for congestive heart failure) was on the telecast as well. The broadcast also featured a photo of me with Senator Grassley and my before and after transplant photos.

The Lord has provided me with free travel to spread the word of adult stem cell research and tell my story. When people argue with me, I like to ask them, "How many adult stem cell transplants have you had?"

Chapter 32: Jolly Ole England

I was so eager to visit our friends in England as many had been praying for me. I missed them and was eager to share my story in person. When we boarded the plane for England, Bill and I went to the back middle section of the plane and, as there were not that many passengers, we took rows of four seats and made beds. A male flight attendant saw my adult stem cell survivor badge and stopped to talk. He congratulated me on my survival. Three female flight attendants sat down beside me and we discussed adult stem cell and embryonic stem cell research. I told my story, Doug's story and gave out Doug's and Dr. Zannos Grekos' e-mails and addresses, as one attendant's father-in-law has congestive heart failure.

At a theatre in London, some people from Canada, who were sitting behind us, read my shirt. They tapped me on the shoulder and told us their neighbor discovered the adult stem cell by accident in 1998. An elderly woman asked about the writing on my shirt also.

Bill and I were enjoying lunch at the Texas Embassy, London when the manager, Thom, sat down with us and congratulated me on my adult stem cell transplant. He was on the National Health list and must wait three years before he would know if they would allow him to have the adult stem cell transplant treatment for his heart. I gave him Doug's information as well as Dr. Grekos. When we paid our bill the cashier informed us that the manager had paid for our margaritas. The last thing he said to me as he hugged me was, "Keep wearing that shirt." I was concerned that if the United States went the way of government controlled health care many would be in Thom's predicament -- waiting to see if the government would allow you to have treatment. Later, at St. James Tavern, Piccadilly Circus, a couple from Wales sat next to us and we talked. He also told me to "keep wearing the shirt."

When we arrived at Cheltenham Spa, Gloucester, where we stayed with friends for a few days, I received an e-mail from the Family Research Council, Washington, DC. confirming I was to be part of a panel on Friday, May 11, 2007 with a pastoral and FRC panel on stem cell research.

Bill and I rode to Cardiff, Wales, then on to the St. Fagan Museum of Welsh Life. Leslie, a British Christian, and a man from Zimbabwe stopped me to "chat me up," as the Brits would say. Her trip to London had been cancelled and it was a God-incidence for us to be right where we were. As she spoke to me, I felt filled with peace and knew she was an instrument of the Lord. She spoke to me of hope and encouragement from the Lord. We took the train to Bursledon to visit and stay with Yvonne, a dear friend and prayer partner and part of my rag-tag army of adult stem cell supporters and helpers.

While attending St. Leonard's Church in Bursledon with Yvonne, the Vicar had me explain, during the service, my adult stem cell transplant. Peter, the Vicar, explained that I was an advocate for adult stem cell research which did not destroy innocent embryos. He prayed prayers of protection for me and my advocacy. After the service, at the coffee hour, many people asked me questions.

As Bill and I were walking in Lymington, which is in the New Forest, a woman clerk thought my shirt was supposed to be a joke. I explained the differences between adult and embryonic stem cells. In England, as in the USA, most people only hear or read of embryonic stem cells, the ones that to my knowledge have not saved lives. Everything was going well until I twisted my foot and began limping rather badly. I hoped it was not broken again but determined woman that I was, I kept going. Cancer did not make me weaker but stronger!

We had lunch at the Royal Oak Tavern, Winchester, which is the oldest bar in England, built around 1000 during the reign of Queen Emma and King Ethelred who lived above it. Our waitress had lots of questions pertaining to adult stem cells as I had yet another of my shirts on. That evening we attended the movie *Amazing Grace* at the Harbour Lights Theatre. It was about William "Wilbur" Wilberforce who helped get slavery abolished in Great Britain and its colonies. He died in 1833 and in 1834, abolition was achieved. I learned that a slaver named John Newton became a preacher and wrote the hymn *Amazing Grace*. Women in the theatre lobby asked about adult stem cells so I gave them my cards to check out my website and facts. I found the story of Wilberforce inspiring as he never gave up on his mission -- nor will I.

Yet another day, we had lunch at The Buttery, Chichester. Patrons at the restaurant read my badge and asked about adult stem cells. As we left The Buttery, I laughed when I saw my first three-wheel car in Chichester.

On our way to spend some more time in Windsor, we first drove to Red Funnel Dock and watched ships in the harbour. As we drove out, on the road was painted Dead Slow, meaning drive slooowly. I loved the way Brits word stuff! As we were having lunch in the Black and White Pub, a woman from Rochester, New York asked me about adult stem cells. I was surprised to have another tourist ask me questions as most of my questions usually come from

British subjects.

On Easter Sunday, at St. Leonard's Church (built in 1204), I was prayed over by Suzie and Colin who gave me the message, "Do not worry about your son Daniel. I have not forsaken Daniel and Daniel has not forsaken me." They said my eyes reflected my deep relationship with the Lord. On our way back to Yvonne's home, we saw many black and white colored magpies flying around, and all I could think of was the nursery rhyme I learned as a child about magpies.

Bill, Yvonne and I then visited David and Lesley on Hayling Island. We toured the island and were surprised at how large it was the farm lands, the WWII reinforcements and the beaches made of sand or shells. We ate at the Maypole Inn where I was asked to explain adult stem cells to a woman who chuckled when she read my badge. At first I ignored people who chuckled, but then I came to realize it was ignorance. So after that realization, I began to venture right up to the chuckling people. I mentioned that I saw them laughing and pointing at my shirt, and explained my shirt meant adult stem cells saved my life -- which was not funny but joyous. They usually got flustered but then wanted to know more.

Chapter 33: Busy, Busy and Busier

On April 11, 2007, as we went through security for our flight home, I left my passport in the bin. When I returned to get it, the security officer asked if I would give him a card for information on adult stem cells as he had read my shirt. Of course I gave him a card. As I boarded the plane, a male flight attendant asked about my shirt, too. I explained and gave him my card. Two other flight attendants said to me that President George Bush was against stem cell research. I said he was against embryonic stem cell research, both on ethical grounds and because it doesn't work. The President fully supported the one that worked, which was not embryonic. I felt badly that we had no more time to talk as they were working.

Once home, with snow and then rain and 44 degrees, I had 300 e-mails to go through. One of them was from David Freddoso. He used my experience with Schumer in Washington, DC in an article for the *National Review* but changed my area and didn't use my name because he was unable to get in touch with me. I read it on nationalreview.com and called him. He told me Schumer declined to comment. Hmmm! I also heard from Feminists Choosing Life; we were to meet at the Liberty Café at 10:30 AM as our appointments with assemblymen began at 11.

Another e-mail was from Chris. "Dear Carol, I met you at the Binghamton airport on March 20. You were on your way to London and I was flying back to Santa Monica, California. I complimented you on your adult stem cell tee-shirt and you came over later to chat. I was telling you about my friend out here in Santa Monica who had Parkinson's disease. You thought adult stem cells might help him and you gave me your card. He wishes to talk to you if that is possible. His condition has deteriorated. You could be his best hope. Thank you, Chris." This would be one of the first replies I sent.

In the mail that came while I was in England I found a book, *Beyond Leukemia: The Conclusion to a 10-Year Story of One Man's Cord Blood Miracle* by Stephen Sprague. He wrote on the inside flap, "To Carol 3/15/07 from one patient-advocate to another....keep up the good work! You tell a sincere and convincing story of hope."

I also received thank you letters from Maryland Catholic Conference and Maryland Right to Life, Inc. "Dear Carol, Thank you so much for coming to Annapolis, MD and testifying in support of adult stem cell research. Your story is remarkable and we were so thrilled that you were able and willing to share it with MD legislators (as well as anyone else who saw your tee-shirt)! I wish you and your lovely husband the best. It was a pleasure to meet you both. Warm regards, Cathy McL."

Owego Town Councilman Don Castellucci Jr. wrote, "I saw the *Pennysaver* this week and wanted to send a note. I mentioned you and the cause at my annual dinner. If I can be of any help let me know and I will try to be of assistance. God Bless and you are in my prayers. Sincerely, Don." He and his family wrote, "Carol, we hope this card finds you feeling better. Keep up the fight. You are doing work for future generations. God Bless, Don, Vicki, Donald and Lauren."

When I picked up tee-shirts to hand out for the cause of adult stem cells, I noticed on the receipt that Susquehanna Printers had donated the screening and setup fees. The receipt says, "Our donation to adult stem cell recognition and understanding." There were so many wonderful people that helped in my mission of educating on adult stem cells and saving lives. I also received phone calls about a cancer patient named Bill from three different individuals and called Bill to speak with him.

I found out from my doctor that my foot had an incomplete fracture and I had to wear the "boot" again. I stopped in at the *Pennysaver* to pick up the photo they used of me when they wrote about my trip to Washington, DC. Three women on staff asked me about adult stem cell treatments and therapies.

I received a note from a woman named Rose who lived in Anderson, Indiana. The letter said, "Dear Mrs. Franz, I talked with you about stem cell research at the Edelweiss Restaurant in Staunton, Virginia. I certainly know a lot more after speaking to you. One of the first items in our local paper when we arrived home was this picture I am enclosing of Annie, a quadriplegic, who was leaving the country to receive a $45,000 adult stem cell operation. It seemed that I was meant to learn from you so I could understand what she had to do to even find someone to try to help her. Why do we have to leave the USA? Thank you for educating me. Rose." I replied to Rose that because the FDA had not approved adult stem cell treatment for spinal cord injuries, doctors here in the USA guide patients to treatment places overseas. What a shame -- and since the FDA didn't approve the treatment, most insurance would not pay. People I know that have received treatment overseas have used money donated to them or taken out second mortgages. We all need to "bug" our Congressmen until they give up and help because they can't shut us up!

At Broome Oncology I received an infusion of Zometa to strengthen my bones. My blood counts were all good except the platelets, which were low, and that meant I had to be careful of bruising.

It was 37 degrees and snowy, but Bill and I drove to Albany, New York to meet with the Feminists Choosing Life. Bill hung out in the Café as I teamed with Meg to talk with a number of assemblymen. Michael Benjamin (D) or his staff didn't show. Carl Heastie's (D) agreeable staff met with us. David Koon (D) didn't believe our views on violence on pregnant women and fetuses. He said life doesn't begin until birth. I said, "You've obviously never been pregnant and felt the baby kicking you for months." He did say he'd stress extra sentencing for killing of a pregnant woman. Gary Finch (R) was a dear and helpful man as was Joseph Errigo (R). Joseph Morelle (D) and William Scarborough (D) sent members of their staffs to meet with us. William Magnarelli's secretary met with us as he was in session. Several of the Feminists Choosing Life asked me for tee-shirts and we also had a photo shot of most of us together. Bill and I then left for Owego and arrived home about 7:30. It was a long day but satisfying.

John Kennedy from Sirius Satellite Radio called and we set up an interview for April 25, 2007 at 7:30 AM. Bill Schneeberger and I set up an interview to be simulcast on www.1360wwow.com on May 2 from 10 to 11 AM. Doris Camp and I made arrangements for my presentation at the VFW Post 1431.

Laura, the NP from my transplant team was concerned about my platelet count. If it got too low, I'd need platelet transfusions. She said my sinus and allergy problems may lower platelets and that Bill had to get me to a better breathing place with no pollen. Hooray, this was something I said to him all the time and now it was confirmed by the medical profession. New York State has too many plants, trees, mold, fungus and mildew to be good for my breathing.

I picked up several more shirts reading, "Adult stem cells saved my friend's life" and handed them out. When I dropped one off to my friend, Rose, she said that her friends told her embryonic stem cell research was best. I told her to ask them who they knew that was ever helped with embryonic stem cell research. I said, "I have been to Washington DC and Albany, and most of the Democrats don't seem to understand the difference between adult and embryonic stem cell research. If they did, they would fund adult stem cell research like they do embryonic." She mentioned Senator Hillary Clinton and I said I couldn't even get her attention. She was pro-abortion and also pro-embryonic research, which go hand in hand.

I saw my buddy, Patti Fitzpatrick, as she was in town from Florida. She came up to me on the street and hugged me. I gave her a fuchsia pink stem cell tee-shirt to wear. Patti prayed over me. Her prayer was quite long, but I remember her saying, "I ask the Lord to provide Carol with health, safety, protection in travels and free places to stay, all her needs like traveling expenses met, that people open up their homes to her, and organizations to meet her needs so that she will carry no burden of expenses. God's people need to hear the message of adult stem cell therapies. We need to keep our Christian brothers and sisters alive to be the 'salt of the earth.' Too many people are dying who don't need to. It is not God's will to remove his workers with death. Times are coming when they will be needed. God made us of stem cells so that doctors can go to our bodies for our help." She blessed me and said nice personal things about me but those didn't stick in my mind.

She asked me to go to Van Horn's Jewelers and speak to Michael. I told Michael my story and gave him my card as well as the names of doctors at Broome Oncology and in Syracuse, because he had a family member ill with cancer. I told him of www.stemcellresearch.org and of Angel Flights out of Corning who transported patients to clinics and hospitals for treatments. I told him the Food and Drug Administration and the National Institute of Health was dragging their feet as far as adult stem cell research funding. I said doctors have told me by 2015 people would still get cancer but would not die from it. I don't want to give people false hope, just hope. I stressed that every stone should be turned over; the patient needs a positive attitude and caregivers need to be positive, too.

I spent all day, April 23, trying to find a ride to Albany for New York State Right to Life Lobbying Day. Dr. David Prentice was the speaker, but I was unable to find transportation or anyone to ride with me. I didn't want to drive alone due to the fracture in my foot.

Bill and I shopped at the P&C Grocery Store. A small child kept looking at me as I was wearing a surgical mask because Bill had just spread chemicals on our lawn and also due to the high pollen count. The child's grandmother read my badge, congratulated me, asked about my transplant and why the controversy. I explained adult, embryonic and cloning before they went on their way. I did mention I was speaking at the VFW on June 3 if she wanted to hear more.

Don Castellucci invited me to sit at his table at the Republican Dinner. Marti Sauerbrey asked for a shirt for Chris, her son who lives in Tennessee. He told his mom he thought about me and prayed for me all the time.

Craig signed on to Sirius and recorded the radio show, Seize the Day. There was an Everyday Hero segment about me, telling my story. I worked on letters that I sent to people about the NHI or National Health Institute and how, in my opinion, they were holding back adult stem cell research due to non-funding.

A friend since ninth grade, Sally Martin, told me she believed God allowed me to get sick so I'd tell everyone about adult stem cell research. Others have said the same to me. God works in mysterious ways. Another person told me that if you want to hear God laugh, tell him your plans. I certainly didn't plan on my life being such as it is. I figured I'd be a "snowbird" enjoying sun, water, good food and good books on a beach somewhere. I believe that the Lord sends into my life those I should help. I must have no fear, for fear died on the cross. Nor will I doubt how to deal with people. God's Wisdom will help them, not any wisdom of mine. Nothing will be too much for me if I rely on my Lord. I must remember LOVE is the greatest gift and I must delight in what the Lord is doing. I believe He is healing me, forming me and sending me forth to educate the world, often one person at a time.

I designed a lime green magnetic sign for the rear of my car bumper that says "Adult Stem Cell Transplant Survivor" and had it made at a shop in Owego. When an idea like that comes to me, I work on it immediately as I believe those ideas are prompted by the Holy Spirit.

By the end of April, I was hurting so badly that I took Tylenol for pain. I was walking like an old cripple. Bill asked how I was and I told him I was going to try to find a place in out West for some of the winter so I don't have to ache from the damp weather in Owego.

Bill Schneeberger, www.1360wwow.com, interviewed me on May 2, 2007 on Living Waters Catholic Radio and sent me a CD. He was the same Bill Schneeberger that promoted and sold BOGO Wines.

I attended St. Patrick's Prayer Meeting and testified about witnessing to the Gatwick Airport Security Guard in London, as well as my testimonies in Washington, DC.

I attended the Republican Party Spring Dinner at the Treadway in Owego. It was a great opportunity to pass out my cards and tell people of the wonders of adult stem cell treatments, research and my story.

The first Saturday of the month, our parish in Owego has an event called "Wine and Dine" after the evening Mass. I took bottles of BOGO wine as my "dish to pass." When the musical group took a break, I went to the mike and explained about the wine and the proceeds towards adult stem cell research. I so want people to be informed, and sometimes I just have to get creative!

Chapter 34: On the DC Circuit Again -- Is Anyone Listening?

On May 9, 2007, Doug Rice, Dr. Prentice, Richard Doerflinger and I met personally with Congressman Daniel Lipinski (D-IL), Congressman Chris Smith (R-NJ), Congressman Bill Sali (R-ID), and Congressman Dr. David Weldon (R-FL). We met with the staff of Congressman Daniel Rohrabacher (R-CA) and Congressman JoAnne Emerson (R-MO). Emerson had us meet with a correspondent, which is the lowest position in her office, in a hallway. The young man became ill hearing our survival stories. Emerson voted for embryonic research even though she had said she would not. Oh well, it was her loss, as she missed out on meeting some great people!

The first thing Congressman Smith brought up was my exchange of words with New York Senator Chuck Schumer. Smith was definitely in my corner and backed me up completely. Smith requested before and after pictures of me for a poster so I had Bill send them via the internet to Smith's office. When Smith asked how I knew so much about stem cell research, I said, "Well, ever since Al Gore invented the internet, I have found lots of research on my computer." Everyone in the room roared with laughter.

Doug, David and I met with first time Congressman Bill Sali of Idaho. He was very enthused about Doug's and my stories and asked us to have our picture taken with him. Usually we were the ones who asked for photo opportunities! After we told him our stories, he said, "I am a man of faith." We discussed how God made our bodies with treatments available within us. We next met with Congressman Dr. David Weldon of Florida, who asked us many personal and medical questions.

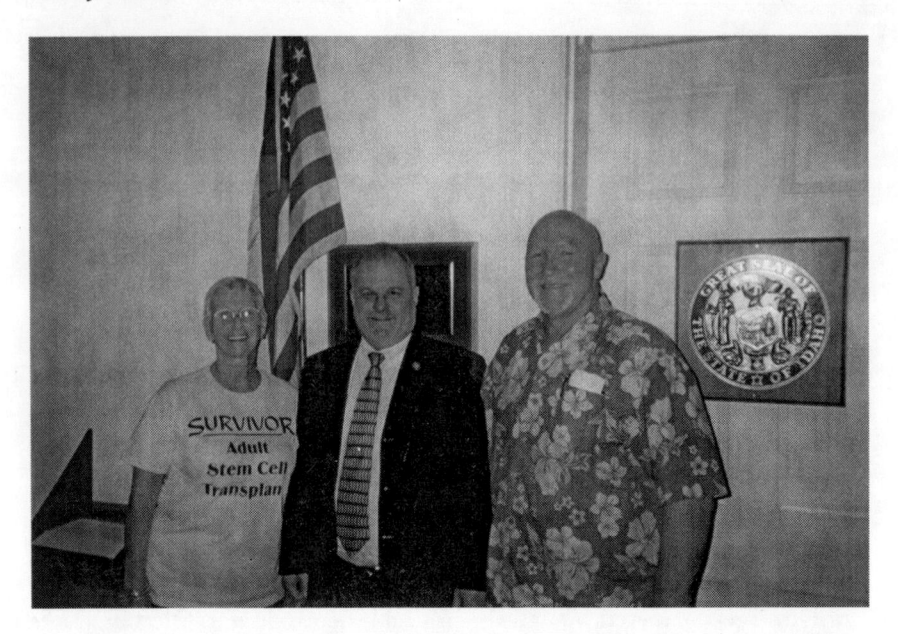

Adult stem cell recipient Doug Rice, Congressman Bill Sali ID (R) and Carol 5/2007

In our cab on the way back from the Hill to the hotel, Doug started talking to our taxi driver, who was Nigerian by birth but was now an American citizen. I told the driver Doug's and my survival stories. The driver started blaming President Bush because he vetoed embryonic stem cell research, so I set the driver straight as I was emboldened by the Holy Spirit. I told him Bush's administration was the only one to fund adult stem cell research and ethical embryonic research as well. I explained why Bush vetoed the embryonic bill and how embryonic research had been funded for many years with no human success stories. The driver said, "You are the only one who has used my cab that had said something good about Bush." I took that in a good way and figured I was better educated than most who rode in his cab!

Doug and I educated a few more cab drivers before our stay in Washington, DC was over. In fact, Doug and I told everyone and anyone we met of our adult stem cell transplants. We even handed out cards to those people who had the opportunity to share elevator rides with us!

As Doug and I were checking out of the Hilton, a woman congratulated me as she read my shirt. I congratulated her right back for knowing about adult stem cell research. Doug and I headed for the Hyatt to check in and then took another cab to Capital Hill. We met up with the others and met personally with Congressman Dr. Phil Gingrey, MD (R-GA) and the staff of Congressmen Buck McKeon (R-CA) and Jason Altmire (D-PA). After lunch we received our official badges and took the underground train to the Capital

There But For the Grace of God

Hill Stem Cell Briefing sponsored by the Do No Harm Coalition, the Family Research Council, the National Right to Life Committee and US Conference of Catholic Bishops. Dr. Weldon, Smith and Lipinski spoke and thanked us for being there. Congressman Smith set up the before and after photo poster of me beside me at the head table. Dr. David Prentice spoke and showed a DVD presentation on stem cell research.

I learned a lot that day! Dr. Prentice talked of studies in the UK and also at the University of Kentucky that used protein GDNF to stimulate the brain to wake up more cells to combat Parkinson's disease. Richard from the Conference of Catholic Bishops also spoke. At the last minute only Congressman Stupak's staff was able to make it – but one of his staff members ordered a tee-shirt from me that said, "Adult stem cells saved my friend's life." Stupak and Lipinski, who in my opinion are two very astute Democrats, were sponsoring a cord blood bill despite their party's push for embryonic research. Apparently they cared more about patients' lives than the party line!

We next attended the VAT or Values Action Team headed by Joe Pitts (R-PA), where Doug and I shared our stories. Dr. Prentice put the huge before and after poster of me up there as well. We asked if there were any questions when we finished our stories. A man from Watertown, New York asked me about the Schumer incident so I told of my experience.

Dr. Prentice and Richard Doerflinger offered Doug and me some of their speaking time at the National Right to Life Convention in Kansas City, Missouri on June 15, 2007. Arrangements were then made by the NRLC for us to speak and have our expenses paid. The Family Research Council would help with our meal expenses. Richard also mentioned keeping August 3, 2007 open, as the Representatives of the Conference of Catholic Bishops would be meeting in Crystal City, Virginia on that date and they would like us to share our stories.

Doug and I returned to the Hyatt to attend the banquet of the Watchmen on the Wall pastors' conference. We received several free booklets, books and DVDs. We shook hands with President Tony Perkins of the Family Research Council and met several other members of the FRC. We were entertained by a Christian comedian, Dennis Swanberg from Texas, and also heard several speeches as well as prayers. Doug was very moved by all of it even though he stated to me that he was not a "religious, church-going man."

Back in my hotel room, I returned a phone call I received from Patty Fitzpatrick in Florida. She had a message from the Lord that I should establish a website and get my book finished and typed as the Lord would use it to assembly an army. I told her I was so busy traveling that it was hard to find the time to type. She said to ask friends for volunteer typists.

When I went to breakfast at the Hyatt, a woman purchased a shirt from me. She paid me $5 over cost and said to use the extra $5 towards a shirt for a person who might not be able to afford it. I have done just that several times over so the extra money helped.

Dr. Prentice, Doug and I spoke to a large number of pastors from all over the USA at the Watchmen on the Wall gathering. I had to leave as soon as our speaking time was completed to catch my flight home. Even so, I was stopped by pastors with questions and requests to speak at their churches. One was Pastor Gary D. Ward of the Rocky Point Baptist Church in Stephenville, Texas who requested a November presentation at his church of several thousand members. Another was Pastor Maria Hunter who gave my card to the parent of a teenager with Non-Hodgkin's Lymphoma. Rev. Posey, whose church was in downtown Atlanta, said he would help get information out on a computer video.

As I rushed through the doors to catch a taxi, the Hyatt doorman, David, exclaimed to me, "I know you. I saw a poster of you when it got carried out of a cab. I was amazed. I need you to answer a question. What is your story?" I explained my story, what adult stem cells are and where they are obtained in the body. I told of other survivors. He called over other employees to listen to me. As I left, in an especially clean cab he obtained for me, David asked if I had ever been on Fox News or CNN. I said, "No, but I'd sure like to." David then replied, "Give me some of your cards. Those guys come here for lunch three or four times a week. The stations are just across the street or around the corner. I'll give them your cards and tell them about you."

During my taxi ride to Dulles, Terry, my taxi driver and I discussed my extension of life due to God, prayer and adult stem cell research. When I arrived at the airport, I found a wheelchair attendant who took me through security, to the bus, and finally to my gate. At every turn, God provided helpers for me getting through the large Dulles Airport easily, as the broken bone in my foot and the "boot" would have slowed me down otherwise. Thanks be to God!

Chapter 35: Have Shirts, Will Travel

Once home, Bill and I drove to Malone to attend Abbey's First Communion. Monsignor Dupree introduced me to Tammy who asked if I would speak to confirmation students in the Fall. Craig set up the website www.carolfranz.com for me, and also made copies of some of my radio interviews so I would be able to send them to his brother and sister. This was also Mother's Day weekend so Terry and Daniel both called.

Back home in Owego, I was exercising at Curves when Gale told me of a staunch Democrat who insisted Gale remove the "Adult Stem Cells Saved My Friend's Life" tee-shirt she had posted, saying the shirt was too political. Gale said it was the truth and the shirt stayed posted on the wall.

At To Your Health food store, Lauren told me when she wore her shirt some people told her that they only knew about embryonic stem cells and doubted her information on adult stem cells. It was so difficult for me to realize how uneducated most Americans were. I wanted them educated before they or a loved one needed help, so they would have the facts about adult stem cell treatments.

I picked up twenty more shirts from Susquehanna Printers and handed them out to friends who desired to help me get the word out. Susquehanna also printed up address cards with my before and after transplant photos on them.

I received phone calls from a person who was suffering from Non-Hodgkin's Lymphoma. They were given my name by a pastor who heard me talk and the person was unaware that people could be treated with adult stem cells for this disease and others. I get so furious that God's people are kept in ignorance by the media, Congress and the pharmaceutical or medical profession on information that might save their lives. Even if people are not candidates for adult stem cell transplant for various reasons, they should still be given the opportunity to investigate all angles to see if it is something that could help them. I have worn these shirts, traveled to speak to groups large and small, and will continue to do so until knowledge gets "out there." I believe I am to take this information and spread knowledge to save souls and lives, and I'll continue until I returned to my Lord.

I received several e-mails, one of which was an invitation to speak at the

National Right to Life Convention on Friday, June 14 along with Doug, Dr. Prentice and Richard. NRLC will pay for my flight and hotel expenses. I accepted.

I heard from Peg, a sister of my friend Mary Dimock. She e-mailed me to let me know that she wore a "friend's life" shirt to all her grandson's baseball games and had been opening eyes in the Victor, New York area. As her granddaughter told her, "You go girl!" Greg, a Vegas friend, wrote to tell me that pro-lifers did not understand adult stem cell research. I told him to spread the word and tell my story. My friend, Anne, sent five DVDs of the TV show we appeared on when I was in Rochester, New York earlier this year.

As Bill and I traveled to Duluth, Georgia for Ty's graduation from high school, I opened my Bible to Acts 28:28: "For the heart of this nation has grown coarse, their ears are dull of hearing and they have shut their eyes." And then there's Isaiah 10:1: "Woe to the legislators of infamous laws." I believe these scriptures fit the USA to a T!

Tyler asked me if there is a God, why does he let kids die and people get cancer? I replied, "I believe it is because of sin. People are made with free will. We are not robots. It isn't God's will, but people cause accidents and sin in the world which attacks the innocent as well as the evil."

Back home, a woman stopped to speak to me after Mass. She said she had been scoping the parishioners and that I was the only one who smiled all during the service. I said, "When you almost die twice, you worship with joy at being alive." I didn't tell her that when the Holy Spirit fills you so completely, joy spills over.

I gave my adult stem cell presentation at the Veterans of Foreign Wars. Avon, Sarah and Kathy manned the tables where I had handouts, photos, tapes and shirts displayed. Joe, photographer for Tioga County *Courier*, took pictures for the paper. The VFW furnished refreshments. The talk went well and the people were dumbfounded at what they did not know about adult stem cell research versus embryonic stem cell research. Little by little I was getting the word out; or rather the Lord was getting the word out via me.

Chapter 36: Carol in the White House, Oh My

A Family Research Council member in DC e-mailed me to see if I could come to Washington on the day President Bush planned to veto the bill that would have endorsed the federal funding of embryonic stem cell research. However, it looked like there would be a conflict with my appearance in Kansas City, Missouri at the National Right to Life Convention. My friends, Candy Gilligan and Sue Motsko, prayed with me at Curves that the timing would work out for both the Kansas City trip and the Washington, DC trip. How nice to have prayerful friends and leave circumstances in the Hand of God!

God constantly puts people in my path that could benefit from knowledge of adult stem cells. When I purchased plants and flowers for my garden and yard, I met a woman who used to live next door. Her son was paralyzed so I sent her information on spinal cord injury and adult stem cell transplants.

I asked my buddy, Walt Beardslee, if he would drive me in the Strawberry Festival Parade with signs on his convertible that said Adult Stem Cell Survivors. I also had a couple of other women interested in joining me -- Louise whose husband survived Myelodysplasia syndrome-leukemia and Mary Lou Robinson who survived multiple myeloma, all with adult stem cells! When dining at the Parkview, I met a woman who donated her bone marrow adult stem cells to her sister Linda who was a cancer survivor. At a Leukemia, Lymphoma and Myeloma Society meeting, I met five adult stem cell survivors and told them to watch for survivors in the parade.

WOW! Bill answered the phone to hear, "This is the White House calling." I'm so glad he didn't hang up on them thinking it was Pete, his high school buddy, playing tricks again. An intern asked me to be at the White House when President Bush made his remarks on stem cell research. He asked for the names of other adult stem cell survivors who would endorse adult stem cell research and might also be interested in attending. I gave him Doug's contact information as well as Mary Lou Robinson's, and told him I'd like to attend. So much was happening so fast. I even received a copy of a *National Review* article from the author who mentioned me together with other adult cell transplant survivors.

June was busy, busy, and busier. Petie Meyers and I went to the Franklin Graham Festival at Binghamton University. I gave my card to the people sitting next to me and discussed adult stem cell research with them. The fellow said it was joyful to see me worship and sing as I radiated joy. On my way out of the festival a young man approached me when he saw my shirt. Rich was from near Cooperstown and had an adult stem cell transplant for leukemia in Boston. I got home to read an email from Dr. Prentice saying that President Bush's veto signing had been postponed. That meant that I had no scheduling conflict between the National Right to Life Convention and my trip to Washington, DC! The women at Curves who just prayed about that couldn't believe it when I told them!

As I re-read the following lines in my journal, I don't know if I wrote them or read them somewhere. "People often choose a way of life that comforts the body but grieves the soul. I think these temporary lives of those on earth are not for our body's comfort but for the strengthening of our souls. We should live in a way that benefits our souls." It sounds too profound for me to have written it but then my life was so busy and the Lord does put things on my mind and heart.

Bill and I went to a Celebration of Life, National Cancer Survivors Day celebration in Liverpool, New York. There was a "flower power" theme so we wore loud clothing. Bill and I were given peace symbols and John Lennon sunglasses to wear. I danced standing in one place due to my foot being in a "boot." I passed out Family Research pamphlets and my cards and answered a lot of questions. One woman used the wording embryonic cord instead of umbilical cord so I explained embryonic versus adult stem cells to her. Many of the nurses didn't realize that adult stem cells are used to treat other diseases besides cancer. One our way home we stopped at Turning Stone Casino and a cashier gave me a "thumbs up" and said, "I believe in adult stem cells." I congratulated her on knowing about them.

Reverend Gary Ward from Stephenville, TX called, inviting me to speak at his church on November. 18. He would pay all my travel expenses as well as Bill's, who was invited to accompany me. Dr. Prentice would be there as well.

My neighbor Rachel Lewis and also Sarah Hall typed some of my book for me as I had so many meetings and engagements. I was blessed to have so many helpful friends. As my schedule filled up, my time to type the book suffered.

Before I knew it, I was on airplane bound for Detroit, Michigan and on to Kansas City, Missouri. I sat next to a man from Denver who asked questions about adult stem cell research due to my shirt. He wanted me to go to Denver to speak as he was a veteran who went to a VA Hospital. Since

There But For the Grace of God

we spoke, the Pentagon had invested money in adult stem cell research and treatments for military personnel.

In the Detroit airport, a woman passed me on the escalator and gave me a "thumbs up" as she read my shirt. While waiting for a tram, a couple approached me and said a friend of theirs was scheduled to have an adult stem cell transplant for multiple myeloma. Could they ask me a few questions? Well, of *course* they could! When clerks asked, "How are you?" I gave them my card. I was a force to be reckoned with. The plane was delayed due to the lack of a pilot, but three women seated near me were also headed to the National Right to Life Convention, and thus I met Melissa, Laurie and Diane. In Kansas City, Missouri, we talked to a young Marine who'd had two tours in Iraq. He told us he was around 1,000 to 2,000 Iraqis every day who were no problem and treated him well. We thanked him for his service. I wish I'd had the time to tell him the Pentagon was using adult stem cells to help our injured military.

Upon arrival at the Kansas City Hyatt, I was met by very enthusiastic Sam Brownback supporters. I had to wait for my hotel room so I checked out exhibits and met NRL Director Jackie Ragan and NRL President Wanda Franz. I met Fr. Frank Pavone of Priests for Life and attended his presentation. 720 babies are aborted and die every hour. People need to hear about this, as they can't imagine an abortion procedure. Legs may be pulled off when the child is taken from the womb. The skull can be brought out in fragments. The child feels pain which is torture. Unthinkable!

In the evening session, we heard messages from President George W. Bush and Fred Thompson. I learned during the General Session that the state of Kansas was reported to be the Abortion Capital of the World. I met Philip Kline, former Attorney General of Kansas who commented favorably on my shirt.

The day started with a Prayer Breakfast where former Congressman Jim Ryan asked for my card and wanted to know if I would ever be able to come to Kansas again to speak. I replied, "Anytime." Janet from Morrill, Nebraska asked about me speaking in Nebraska.

Jeanne from Topeka, Kansas and a Missouri fireman named Dave received "friend's" shirts from me. Dave gave me a Missouri fireman shirt to give to my husband, Bill, who is a volunteer fireman in Owego. St. Louis Archbishop Burke received an award and Archbishop Joseph Neumann from Kansas City, KS spoke.

At 12:45 PM, Dr. Prentice, Richard Doerflinger, Doug and I spoke at a workshop entitled "Myths and Realities of Stem Cell Research." It was well-attended and many asked questions. I went to many other workshops wearing my shirt. In all I passed out about 300 cards that showed my before and after photos and listed my website.

The evening ended with a General Session of the Republican Presidential Forum. I heard speeches from Ron Paul, Mitt Romney and Sam Brownback. I shook Mitt's hand and gave him my card. I flew back home before the convention ended as I had commitments in Owego on Saturday.

Walter, Mary Lou, Louise and I rode in a convertible in the Owego, New York Strawberry Festival Parade. People who knew what we represented cheered and clapped their hands. I shouted out to blank faces that adult stem cells from our own bodies saved our lives. Next year I need to get a loudspeaker. Wendy of the *Pennysaver* took our photo. I learned when I arrived home that an intern, Matt, from the White House had called with details on my trip to Washington.

Terry, Molly, Craig and his girls joined Bill and me at Fr. Watt's 50th Jubilee Mass. I greeted folks and gave out programs. During the service Pat Burnett sat behind me. I told her about my invitation to the White House. She offered her son Dan's help as he lived near the airport there; she told me Dan would probably put me up so I wouldn't have to rent a hotel room or a car. Later at the reception I talked with Dr. Michaels and thanked him again for saving my life by diagnosing my cancer. He told me he had a copy of the *Morning Times* article about me framed on his office wall. He said it was not every day that a rheumatoid arthritis doctor got thanked for saving someone's life.

When I got home, I received a printed invitation via e-mail for the White House proceedings and a phone call from Dan Burnett, my friend Pat's son, who extended an invitation to stay at his family's home while I was in DC. Dan was one of the teenagers who spent Sunday evenings at our home for the Christian Awareness Program. He also was delighted when we named our new son Daniel, and gave us a wall hanging for Dan's room that he and his mom had made. It had been years since we had seen each other but he was willing to help his First Communion teacher. God bless him. He was a joy. That was a God-incidence for sure.

I purchased my airline ticket for Washington DC, and as it was short notice the cost was $698.80. I put it on our charge card and when I told Bill and Terry they questioned who was paying. I told them an organization but I didn't know which one. The Lord said He would provide all my needs. They kept harping on it but I knew in my heart it would be repaid by God's helpers somehow.

I received another call from Matt the intern, saying I'd be on the dais behind President Bush when he gave his remarks on stem cell research. I would also have a private photo op in the Green Room of the White House where I would have the opportunity to speak with the President personally. I was

There But For the Grace of God

taking it in stride, but the friends I told were really psyched and excited about my adventure. Someday maybe my great- grandchildren will be impressed that I spoke with the President of the USA in the White House!

As I was getting ready to go to the airport, I received a phone call from a new friend that lived about 90 miles from Owego. She asked how I was paying for my ticket and how much it was. I told her I had used our credit card. She said, "I am sending you a check for $700 to cover your flight expenses. If another group offers to pay, please accept them graciously and put my money under the mattress or something. Use it to supplement the tee-shirts/sweatshirts and incidentals associated with your activities. Bless you for what you are doing!" I made sure Bill and Terry heard this news!

As I arrived at the Washington DC airport, the *Binghamton Press & Sun-Bulletin* called me on my cell to interview me then and there by the luggage pickup. Dan found me and cooked supper for me and his family. Neither Dan nor his wife Kristen knew about stem cell research differences or therapies but they sure do now. I called Dr. Prentice and confirmed that it would be all right for me to hang out in his office at the Family Research Council as Dan would drop me off there on his way to work. Dr. Prentice and Richard of the Conference of Catholic Bishops wished to share in paying my flight expenses. I told them someone had already offered, but they said to use that money for other expenses. I made sure Bill and Terry heard this news as well!

And suddenly, oh my -- it was June 20, 2007, the day I was to meet the President of the United States. But first, when I arrived at the Family Research Council, Doug, Dr. Prentice and I took a cab to a Democrats for Life meeting. (Who knew?) Dr. Prentice showed slides of me during his scientific presentation, after which I gave my personal story. Doug told his story as well. Afterwards we all answered questions. The people had known very little of what we were speaking about and were amazed at what had been accomplished in adult stem cell research and therapies. We also met a young student at the College of Steubenville, Ohio whose mother was a ten-year survivor of breast cancer with the help of an adult stem cell transplant. The three of us presenting were excited to hear of another adult stem cell survivor. It was always so uplifting and humbling to be able to share hope and success with people who were unaware of adult stem cell research. We left there and rushed directly to the White House.

Chapter 37: President George W. Bush Meets Determined Carol Franz

I had to be at the White House earlier than the other adult stem cell survivors as I had a gift for President Bush and needed to give it to the Secret Service to inspect. My gift was a tee-shirt made by Susquehanna Printers of Owego that said, "Adult Stem Cells Saved My Friend's Life." I informed the President's staff that I had also sent President Bush a shirt at his address in Crawford, TX. They said they would check on that shirt right away. Everyone was very kind, patient and friendly.

I was escorted through security and into the White House as all the other survivors, visitors and attendees went in by another way. I had my own intern who accompanied me, explaining what would be happening, such as waiting for the President in the Blue Room for a private photo op and visit. I was allowed to roam in the Green Room and the Red Room. The rooms are just that. The color is the predominate theme of the carpet, walls, draperies and furniture. The Blue Room reminded me of rooms that I had seen and been in at Buckingham Palace in London.

While I waited for the President I wandered into the Green Room which was where the politicians and other survivors were waiting. I introduced Mary Lou Robinson to many Senators and Congressmen as well as to other survivors. I had submitted Mary Lou's name to the White House and they invited her to attend. We all paid our own expenses. People might be glad to know that taxpayer dollars did not subsidize any of us.

A rehearsal was staged so that we would know where to stand on the dais. I noticed seats with names on them and suggested to an aide that one be saved in the front row for the Texan adult stem cell survivor as I was sure the President would like the Texan front and center. That worked out well for Doug, who was living in Texas at the time -- and for me, as he had borrowed my camera! Soon everyone left the Green Room to fill the seats in the East Room, which soon filled up with other adult stem cell transplant survivors, Congressmen and newsmen. I stayed behind in the Blue Room with my Air Force and Marine escorts. Kaitlyne McNamara, an eighteen-year-old born with spina bifida, and her family were also there. We were seated at different sides of the room and awaited the President. Kaitlyne had her own adult stem cells removed from her diseased bladder and those cells were used to create a new bladder for her in a Wake Forest laboratory by Dr. Anthony Atala. The new bladder was then put into her body which saved her life.

We were all filled with joy but not nervous. It was a happy time for us. President Bush came strolling in and visited first with the McNamara family, hugging Kaitlyne and greeting each family member. They visited and had a photo shot.

Then it was my turn. President George W. Bush and I stood side by side as he shook my hand and congratulated me on my adult stem cell transplant and surviving cancer. I gave him my card which includes my before and after photos. He put on his glasses to look at it and I asked if he wanted me to stand in front of him to shield him from a photo shot in his eyeglasses. We both laughed and then I gave him his "tee-shirt" and said it represented over 400,000 people treated with adult stem cell transplants. I told him I have over 60 friends wearing these shirts in 22 different states and 3 foreign countries. The photographer took a photo of us with the President holding the shirt in front of us. President Bush then gave it to an aide and we proceeded to have another photo. He put his arm around me and I asked if I was allowed to put my arm around him; he said, "Yes, of course."

We then walked hand in hand in the room and visited. I told him I came from Tioga County, New York, which voted Republican even though the counties around us and our state didn't. I told him we are a pro-life county. I also mentioned that prior to the 2004 November elections, I was on local television giving the story of my adult stem cell transplant and the end table near me had his photo on it, and that photo appeared in the television coverage. On the broadcast I explained that the Bush administration was the only administration to finance adult stem cell research and that he was pro-life. I informed the President that many local people told me that they changed their minds and voted for him because of that interview. He replied, "Thank you and I am so happy you are well. Keep up the good work." There were other words between the President and me as well. I was as comfortable with him as I am my dearest friends. I was very relaxed and at ease with President Bush and it was very obvious to my inner spirit, what a man of faith he is.

I had quite an experience on June 20, 2007. I was privileged to stand with George W. Bush, President of the United States of America, as he made remarks on stem cell research and vetoed the bill S5 which would have funded, with tax dollars, only embryonic stem cell research. The President did not outlaw embryonic stem cell research. It was legal and happening across the nation. What President Bush said was that Congress shouldn't fund destructive research with our taxpayer dollars, especially when promising alternatives exist. The power of adult stem cell research has the power to save lives, as it did mine. We shouldn't be destroying some people's lives to save the lives of others.

We all cheered and clapped for a long time. During the clapping and cheering, I whispered, "Thank you" to the research doctor next to me. Dr. William Hurlbut congratulated me on my recovery. The clapping and cheering stopped and the President continued his speech. In his speech he said, "I'm also up here with Carol Franz; she has whipped cancer twice by using adult stem cells....She's a determined woman who believes strongly that there are different alternatives available to use stem cells other than those which are created as the result of destruction of human life." He also told about Kaitlyne and kept hugging her or patting her head as he was emotionally taken by her story. President Bush then issued an executive order promoting the funding of all pluripotent stem cell research which includes all adult stem cell research. This research was an ethical alternative to embryonic stem cell research and did not harm human life as embryonic did. I was grinning from ear to ear and folks were again clapping very loudly.

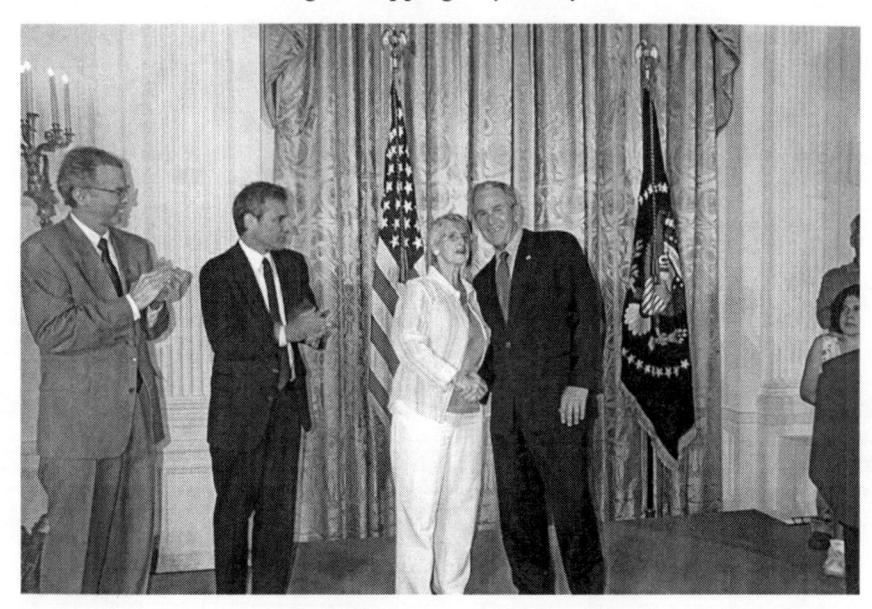

Dr. D. Landry, Columbia Univ., Dr. W. Hurlbut, Stanford Univ., Carol Franz, President G. W. Bush, Kaitlyne McNamara and father; White House East Room on June 20, 2007

At the end of his speech, the President turned, grasped my hand and talked some more to me. I whispered in his ear that a fellow Texan seated in the front row was an adult stem cell survivor for congestive heart failure and diabetes. The President went down the steps and shook Doug's hand. After the ceremony I happily spent a great deal of time shaking hands with politicians, pastors, newscasters, other survivors and visitors. I was not nervous as all these people sought me out. I got the idea that being included in the President's gathering made people take notice of me when they otherwise might not. I thanked the Lord for giving me this opportunity.

I considered it an honor for a Christian, Catholic woman from the tiny village of Owego, in upstate New York to have had the opportunity to meet the President of the United States of America, George W. Bush as well as be a witness for the saving power of adult stem cell research.

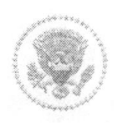

THE WHITE HOUSE

WASHINGTON

July 24, 2007

Mrs. Carol Franz
257 Prospect Street
Owego, New York 13827

Dear Carol:

It was an honor to have you at the White House. Your story is a wonderful example of how stem cells can be used to help those in need while upholding our fundamental moral values. Thank you for letting me share your experience of hope and healing.

Best wishes.

Sincerely,

George W. Bush

Chapter 38: Home Again But Not for Long

I had scarcely gotten home from Washington, DC, before I was contacted by Raymond Arroyo of Eternal Word Television Network, EWTN, World Over Live. Raymond and his son were seated in the front row along with Doug in the East Room, which was how Raymond learned of me. He interviewed me on his TV show live via the telephone. He also interviewed Fr. Tad Pacholczyk, the doctor/scientist/priest whose clear explanation of adult stem cell research and other survivors enlightened so many. Callers around the world responded telling of their successful adult stem cell treatments.

At home several local interviews were requested by the *Morning Times*, Sayre, PA, the *Tioga Courier* and also the *Pennysaver*. I was annoyed that the Binghamton *Press and Sun-Bulletin* didn't use my DC interview but managed to mention me (and the President) in a negative tone. Too bad the liberal media didn't want the public to know the truth about the life saving effects of adult stem cells.

But reactions like that were few. Much more typically, I received emails like "Congrats Carol and thanks for representing the Truth for us. Lord, please raise up more Carols!!! And bless her with all your best today Father. Go Get Em Carol, Cathryn M." (To the best of my knowledge, I've never met Cathryn.)

From Irene in Vegas: "You are doing the Lord's work. God Bless you,"

"Sister Carol, Good Morning. What a blessing you are doing [in your] work for the Lord, [giving] Him the honor, glory and praise. We are so blessed to have had you in our St. Joseph's Las Vegas prayer group. When in town, stop by. The group will keep you in our prayers, please remember us in your prayers. God's blessing, Sister Geneva,"

"Cheers to you Mom. I couldn't be prouder of you. You are an inspiration! I love you dearly, your loving daughter, Terry

"I watched it on TV and words can not express the wonder of it all. God's ways are truly, truly awesome. How amazing that your illness would touch the world! On my face before Him, Fannie."

"Carol, I wanted you to know that I watched the press conference on TV and was so blessed when you whispered in his ear. Many, many thousands more lives will be touched by adult stem cell research, I am sure. I was sharing with a group last evening and not one of them [had] heard of it! May I send your e-mail to me of your trip to Valerie Zehl at the *Press*? Fannie." (I replied, "By all means, please do. I urge everyone I talk to that they should learn about adult stem cell research as the life they save may be their own. I was interviewed over the phone by the *Press* but the editor opted not to print it. This reporter may do it justice. Thank you for your encouragement. P.S. I have at least three more trips in the works in Washington DC. One is a stem cell debate, one is a meeting with representatives of the US Conference of Catholic Bishops and one is an FRC conference with pastors from all over the US and Canada.")

Several people wanted copies of photos of President Bush and me, so I had some made. They hang in businesses and are carried by people who believe in adult stem cell research.

The next day I was coming home after picking up some Adult Stem Cell Survivor bumper stickers I had ordered when I drove past an anti-war group (no one likes war) protesting in Court House Memorial Park. A sign stated LIES KILL LIVES. I stopped the car and went up to the man holding the sign. I told him his sign also represents what I advocate, lies about embryonic stem cell research and lies hiding the success of adult stem cell research, both of which lead to lives lost. As the Book of Isaiah says, people perish for lack of knowledge. People hear about all sorts of entertainment trivia in the media, but no one hears about the 2000 Americans that die each day of congestive heart failure and heart ailments or the 1500 Americans that daily die from cancer within our country's own borders. I told the man I respected his views on war but I don't share them. He had no idea about adult stem cell research, so of course, I filled him in. We thanked each other for our comments and I left.

About an hour later I received a phone call from this gentleman. He had called every Franz in the phone book until one of them gave him my number. He said the other protestors wanted to know about our conversation. When we spoke I was wearing a shirt that said, Former Embryo. He asked if I was the same woman pictured with the President and where he could obtain information, so I sent him to my website, www.carolfranz.com

Renee, a woman I met in a HEB grocery store in Cedar Park, Texas called me from Altoona, Kansas where she actually resided. She had a friend in Oklahoma who was ill and wanted information on clinical trials, so I sent her to my website, told her to go to links, and then click on www.clinicaltrials.gov. When this woman asked her oncologist about adult stem cell transplants, he told her it was too painful and she should wait for embryonic stem cell transplants to be perfected. *What?!?* This doctor was completely ignorant about adult stem cell transplants. Doctors like this one were the reason I encouraged patients to go for second, third, even fourth opinions in order to find an intelligent doctor who practiced up-to-date medicine. Renee said she told everyone about me and asked if she could have a "friends" shirt, so I sent her one.

I googled "carol franz stem cell" and many articles came up. I didn't realize so much was out there about me. Many articles were in foreign countries as well as across the US.

Boy oh boy, was I annoyed with New York Lt. Governor Paterson (now Governor Paterson). I wrote to the *Albany Times* pertaining to a letter from Paterson, printed 6/22/07, which I felt was full of misinformation about stem cell research. Of course, *my* letter was not printed by the paper. I keep thinking people would want to print the truth, but I guess most media "just can't handle it!"

I was with President Bush when he vetoed the act which would have funded only embryonic, not adult, stem cell research. I too am a long time supporter of "SCR" (stem cell research) but I support *adult* stem cell research that actually works and has saved my life as well as the lives of thousands of others. I too have high moral standards but I am not willing to sacrifice some human lives for experiments. How high could his standards be when he pushed research that was known to be scientifically "iffy" and ignored proven research?

And he didn't even express himself accurately. He called embryonic stem cells "the only pluripotent cells in the human body." Embryonic stem cells are not in the body, certainly not in anyone that's born. You have to remove them from an embryo, killing the embryo in the process, to get them "out of the body." His grasp of science was poor, ignoring all the numerous pluripotent stem cells now known, including those from bone marrow, cord blood, amniotic fluid, etc. Adult stem cells are regenerative medicine that restore and repair the body. Embryonic stem cells grow a separate living organism. New York State would save lives by funding adult stem cell research. It works now; you don't have to wait for some future time. I personally know people that have been treated with adult stem cells using adult stem cells from their own bodies, cord blood or donors.

Each day I had patients, doctors, family members, and friends who called me for information about adult stem cell treatments for congestive heart failure, damaged organs, and cancers of all kinds. I handed out my cards and answered e-mails and phone calls but stressed that I was not a doctor or scientist -- just a recipient survivor whose life was returned to her through adult stem cell treatment. I told everyone to go to www.carolfranz.com which had several links that would give information in detail on adult stem cell research and clinical trials. Do No Harm has posted a You Tube address called "stemcellsthatwork" and have posted videos of me and other stem cell survivors. http://www.youtube.con/stemcellsthatwork

I brag about Texas because for the first time in their history, their state budget had millions of dollars for treatments and research using adult stem cells. All funding for human cloning and embryonic stem cell research, which destroyed human embryos, was pretty much stopped. The legislature was funding the collection of cord blood at hospitals across Texas and storing those adult stem cells in a public bank such as the Texas Cord Blood Bank at *no* cost to the birth mothers. These adult stem cells would be available for treating patients with diseases such as cancer or sickle cell anemia. More money would go toward research to find more treatments at research institutes. I have friends from many states that have gone to Texas for treatment, because Texas is concentrating on saving lives now.

For years millions of dollars had been spent on embryonic research at the expense of saving lives with funding for adult stem cell research. I've heard there will be clinical trials for diabetes held in Waco during 2009. Texas has done clinical trials for the heart and other diseases. I have met many Texans who were unaware of all of this, thanks to some of their liberal newspapers.

I have told my story to:

- National Right to Life Conventions
- US Conference of Catholic Bishops Secretariat for Pro-Life Activities
- St. Helen's Church, Georgetown, TX
- The Washington Briefing, Values Voters Summits
- Radio interview by Shelly Wynter 1380 AM WAOK
- Binghamton Seratoma Club;
- Broome County Priests Meeting
- Our Lady of Angels Church Confirmation Classes
- Malone, NY Catholic Confirmation Classes
- Ave Maria Radio
- Right to Life, Life-Span, Livonia MI
- Rocky Point Baptist Church, Stephenville, TX
- St. Mary's Assumption Church, Waco, TX
- St. Stephen's Church, Salado, TX
- Bishop Gorman High School, Las Vegas, NV

...And others that are listed on my website, www.carolfranz.com, as well as links to sites that will help with information on where clinical trials are being held.

Epilogue

I basically wrapped up the writing of this book in 2007. But it's now 2009, and of course things have continued to happen.

My husband, Bill has grown to be an even more tremendous help and support for me.

In 2008 I was videotaped for You Tube, thus using the internet to provide students from around the USA with information they can use when writing their term papers on adult stem cell research. A new video with other adult stem cell survivors and me will be released on You Tube in 2009.

I met Barry Goudy, a five-year survivor of MS using his own adult stem cells.

I gave my card to Michael Medved, Star Parker, Carl Rove, Sen. Fred Thompson, Rep. Chris Smith, Michael Steele, Coach Joe Gibbs, and Ken Wales, who produced the movie *Amazing Grace*. I've also given my card and my testimony to hundreds of strangers that I have encountered. I've been interviewed by Tony Beam of Christian World View Today, Rom Bogart of the North Dakota Catholic Radio, and the Indiana Right to Life radio.

I gave presentations at Coalition for Moral Cancer Research in Norcross, Georgia and at the Kentucky Right to Life Convention held in Louisville, Kentucky. I am booked to give workshops at National Right to Life Convention in Charlotte, North Carolina, Pennsylvania Pro-Life in Scranton, Pennsylvania and Values Voter Summit in Washington DC so far this year.

I wrote to Mike Huckabee and asked him to have adult stem cell survivors on his TV show to get the word out to patients and doctors. I am waiting to hear from him.

I also wrote many letters to newspapers around the country, as well as members of Congress.

I learned of more success stories with adult stem cell treatments, such as a woman obtaining a new windpipe using her own bone marrow and a donated trachea.

I joined five other adult stem cell survivors in handing out information on adult stem cells to a crowd of 20,000 people attending the 2008 Owego Strawberry Festival. Some of the adult stem cell transplant recipients walked and others rode in a car in the parade.

Carol J. Franz

At the 2008 Tioga County Fair, my friends and I asked for signatures on petitions to establish an umbilical cord blood bank in upstate New York – a measure which was passed by past Gov. Pataki, but dropped by then-Gov. Spitzer and Gov. Paterson. Our petition stated that whereas over $600 million in taxpayer funds have been committed over the coming years to New York State stem cell research; and whereas New York State Chapter 427 of the Laws of 2007 require education and outreach on the benefits of cord blood banking; and whereas those born and raised in upstate New York State have similar tissue types; and whereas the 2007-2008 New York State Budget committed money to the "design and construction of an umbilical cord blood bank facility"; and whereas upstate New York has no universal public cord blood bank, we the undersigned request that an upstate New York universal cord blood bank facility be established soon to provide cord blood information and storage to upstate patients.

A federal bill was passed in December 2005 that every state should establish cord blood banks for free storage of cord blood by birth mothers, which in turn can be used universally for anyone who needs the blood for an adult stem cell transplant. Most cords can hold enough blood to help up to four patients, yet many states ignore helping their citizens this way. Four thousand babies are born in the USA each year and most of the cords are thrown away as medical waste. I am hoping citizens all over the United States will start "bugging" their state's politicians to get busy establishing adult stem cell umbilical cord blood banks.

On August 8, 2008 I was again determined to be in relapse with my third session of Multiple Myeloma. Today, in 2009, I am taking Thalomid to destroy the cancer cells. I have one vial of adult stem cells still frozen at Upstate Medical in Syracuse. I travel, give presentations, and do all that I have done in the past to further spread knowledge of adult stem cells. In 2003, my doctors told me they would keep me alive for the day when a cure for cancer is found. Praise God for only He knows the numbering of my days. I try to live as joyously as I can each and every day. I have told friends not to accept a doctor's numbering of their days.

I learned, from a retired IBM nurse attending one of my workshops, that Dr. Judson, who lived in Endicott area but worked at Owego and Glendale IBM in the late 1950's invented one of the first blood separator machines. His son had died from leukemia so Dr. Judson asked IBM for a leave of absence to do research. Instead IBM paid for Dr. Judson's research and he continued working. The nurse informed me that every six months the staff received gamma globulin which protected the nurses from infection because the nurses worked with bad blood. My husband informed me that several IBM workers donated blood to be used in this research.

I had heard of Dr. Judson before but never met anyone who knew him personally or worked with him. The first machine that sorted adult stem cells was invented by a local IBMer. To me that is so cool!

I have persevered in telling my story as I did when I met Paris Hilton, Siegfried and Roy, Jamie Farr, and Frankie Avalon during my time in Las Vegas. I believe my mission is to educate all those I meet, because a higher power than myself is leading me.

I am still being contacted by people who have either met me by chance, heard me speak, or visited my website. They tell me how encouraging and hopeful it is to learn about adult stem cell therapies for so many illnesses or disabilities. An example is from Vesna Gasovska who lives in Macedonia, a small European country. "Dear Carol, Thank you so much for the information. I highly appreciate it. Honestly, I didn't expect that you would answer me at once and send me a lot of information that would help me. God is there for every one of us. I got answers from Prof. McGuckin in Paris, France, Dr. Kurtzberg at Duke University and Dr. Baumgartner about the possibilities of treating my daughter, Ana Gabeloska, someday with adult stem cell cord blood, for her cerebral palsy. Thank you, Carol, so much. I would have never had this information without your help."

I can be contacted at www.carolfranz.com to answer questions, or if more information is needed about adult stem cell therapies and clinical trials. I have access to many doctors and scientists involved in adult stem cell research that I contact before sending the information. As I said before, I am not a doctor or scientist but one who is alive due to God's Grace and some knowledge of adult stem cell therapies. Many doctors and nurses do not have up-to-date information.

Second Corinthians 12:9 reads: "My grace is sufficient for you, for power is made perfect in weakness." Without the weakness of experiencing cancer and adult stem cell transplants, I would not have had the ability to be invited to Washington, DC to the White House, give many talks on Capital Hill, and speak on Eternal Word Television Network, the National Right to Life Conventions, the Voter Values Forum or any of the numerous groups and people I have encountered. I believe God has chosen me despite my weakness and made manifest His will. None of us are perfect but by God's Grace I persevere. Second Corinthians 12:10: "for the sake of Christ; for when I am weak, then I am strong."

Blessed and glad to be alive,
Carol J. Franz

References and Sources

Carol Franz journals

[1, 5, 6, 7, 8] *The Word Among Us*. Reprinted with permission of *The Word Among Us*, 9639 Dr. Perry Rd. # 126, Ijamsville, MD

King James Bible

[2, 3, 4] *Living Faith, Creative Communications for the Parish*, LF Books, 1564 Fencorp. Dr., Fenton, MO, Philadelphia, and New York reprinted with permission

EWTN, Birmingham, Alabama

Rick Burt stem cell explanation letter

Jane Doty letter

E-mails from Margaret, Emy, Kathy Bachman, Irene, Jane, Doug, Kathy.

Terry's letter for contest of Godmother of the Seas

Marie's note

Carol's letter to Laura Bush

Phil's letter

Most Rev. Joseph A. Pepe's, Bishop of Las Vegas, NV letter

Fr. Charles Van Winkle's letter

Most Rev. Arroyo, Bishop of Austin, TX letter

First Lady Laura Bush's letter to Carol

www.stemcellresearch.org, Do No Harm 1100 H. St. NW., Suite 700. Washington, DC 20005

www.clinicaltrials.gov Washington, DC

Carol's letter to grandson, Tyler

Yvonne's letter from England

Adrian's letter

Sandy Solomon's note

Jo S. letter

Jane Doty's note

Busch Garden worker's letter

Feminists Choosing Life letter

Chris M letter

Rose B. letter

1360www.com radio/computer interview

Patti's prayer

DC Circuit

Encounter with Senator C. Schumer

Peg's e-mail

National Right to Life Convention 2007

Meeting President Bush

White House Photo by Doug Rice

Book Cover photos by Bill Franz, Craig Franz, and Kathy Bergmann

Congressman Bill Sali photo with Doug Rice and Carol Franz by Bill Franz

E-mails from friends on White House visit

Anti-war group in Owego, NY

Letter to Lt. Gov. Paterson

Siegfried and Roy

Paris Hilton

Frankie Avalon

Jamie Farr

www.carolfranz.com containing links to adult stem cell research sites

Letters of Encouragement

I received over 700 letters and e-mails as well as several Mass cards during my illness and recoveries. A few samples are included here.

"Carol,

I tried to stay calm when I talked to you on the phone, even though I didn't feel it inside. You are very special to me. I can't begin to tell you how your health crisis has affected me. I am enclosing the prayers I talked to you about. The Larry Hess Prayer we prayed years ago. The St. Peregrine Prayer, Jim and I are saying every day and sending the same out to other prayer warriors that have asked for it. Know we are standing with you. We know Bill and Carol are strong people and know the Lord is watching over you. Love you guys -- Jim & Sandy."

"Just want to let you know that you are in my prayers. I still want you to know, I wake up in the middle of the night. I ask God to be with whoever needs prayer at that time. I hope you feel them when you are in need. Sometimes I know who he wants me to pray for and other times I don't. I learned from Father Tom that I should pray anyway. I am sure that you have done that for years. You are one of my favorite examples of a prayer intercessor.

Love, Joan Kenderish."

"Dear Mrs. Franz,

I am so sorry to hear of your illness and hope that you are getting through your treatments, procedures and care, on the way to recovery. We are all thinking of you. You and your family are in our prayers. I have been thinking of you lately -- and with that --fondly remembering how you and Mr. Franz were such warm and wonderful leaders of our Teen Religious Christian Awareness Program or CAP Group. I wonder how you two were so brave (especially because now I have teens, and I help out with our youth group at our church). I remember you ALWAYS feeding us—especially building ice cream sundaes at your home. I also remember our Teen Group trip to the Washington Mall, and also a retreat over one weekend. Now I can really appreciate all you both did for us because I help out with our youth group. So, a BIG thank you. We will continue to pray for you and your family.

God Bless, Love, Joanie Meyers Delaney."

Belfort, France

"Dear Carol and Bill,

Please accept our best wishes of joy, happiness and good health. May 2003 bring you good health, especially for Carol and for all your family. Much rest and courage are needed for the treatments are long, but Carol is very strong and this will be a hard moment for you but I think you will be better soon. Thank you for your warm wishes and your photo. Now I will have a souvenir of my American cousins. All of the family and me send you kisses,

Christiane Nowak."

Bursledon, Southampton, England

"Carol dear, let me hold your hand right now. 'The Lord is our helper, we shall not want.' We have a prayer notice board now in the North Transept at St. Leonard's Church near a small cross and candles. Your name is there. Thank you for keeping in touch. St. Leonard's & St. Paul's Take Notice Sheet has a prayer request that Carol Franz respond to stem cell treatment. [It asks people to] please also pray for Carol's husband Bill and family. God Bless you, Carol.

Love from Felix Neville-Towle.

Dear Carol –

How lovely to receive your letter to us. We will be praying for you with our whole hearts as you go through this huge programme of restoration. You are a wonderful example of faithfulness and trust in God because you will need Him each step of the way. He will be with you and with Bill and will give you the strength that you need to face all that lies ahead.

With my love, Jean Neville-Towle,"

Owego,

"My Dear Carol,

For months now, when I do my walk for exercise and prayer, I've been drawn to Prospect St. and thinking of you. This is long before I got the news of your illness. It must be that spiritual closeness we have that you mentioned on the phone when we last spoke. Please be assured of my prayers and great hope for you. My admiration of your strength, courage and positive attitude are even greater than they've always been—which is a lot! You are truly an inspiration to me and many, many others.

Yours always in Christ and Hope, Love, Mike Fowler."

"Carol,

As I have watched you over the last months, going from 'I really don't feel well' to the implanting of the stem cells over a week ago, I can't begin to tell you how much I admire you. Sarah and I were saying on the way home that neither one of us were sure how we ourselves would do in a similar situation. In spite of how ill you felt yesterday, after we prayed together, you wanted to pray for the young man next door. Your caring attitude for others is one of the many reasons we are blessed with having you as our forever friend. Hang in there, Carol. You are in the home stretch.

Love, Sandy Ross."

"Dear Bill and Carol,

Remember a month or so back when I met you guys at Lourdes Hospital? I was shocked and concerned at the physical state Carol was in. Just the other day I was reminded again through conversation with an individual I was talking to. I want you both to know that I don't take such things with an indifferent attitude, but I am concerned and I am praying and trusting in the Lord God My Savior to be with you in this trial.

No one can know the weight that is upon you at this time but He who knows all things, God Himself. Christ said in His word, 'Ye believe in God, believe in me also.' In Matt. 11:28, Christ tells us, 'Come unto me, all ye that labor and are heavy laden and I will give you rest.' And in Vs. 29: 'Take my yoke upon you, and learn of Me for I am meek and lowly in heart; and you shall find rest unto your souls.' Vs. 30: 'For my yoke is easy and my burden light.'

These words may not seem to apply in your situation, but I believe as you lean on Him, He will lighten the load or burden you are carrying. I believe He is able to heal us through whatever course we need to take to accomplish that. Ultimately healing must come from Him. When Christ stood trial and was beaten (lashed), he did it for us in becoming weak that we could be healed. Isaiah 53:5 says 'He was wounded for our transgressions, He was bruised for our iniquities; the chastisement of our peace was upon Him and with His stripes we are healed.' I wanted to point out this scripture as it can apply to your need. The whole chapter of Isaiah 53 about Our Lord suffering is a good word to meditate upon. I haven't meant to preach; I just wanted you to know I'm concerned and want you to know you are not alone in this. I know there is hope. I am praying for you and will continue to do so.

Love in Christ,
Art Reynolds."

Blessed Trinity and Saint Patrick's Parish pastor and parishioners prayed over and blessed a blanket that was requested for me by Keith and Sue Ballard. St. Patrick's Bulletin listed Carol Franz on their Prayer List for my entire illness and recovery time.

"Dear Carol,
    During worship at the United Methodist Church, Empire, Michigan, we dedicated and anointed a prayer cloth for you which is included with this note. Please know that you have lots of prayers coming your way.
    Love,
    Pete and Sandy Mallory."

St. Leonard's and St. Paul's Bursledon, England Take Notice Sheet asked prayers for "Carol Franz, who is responding to adult stem cell treatment. Please also pray for Carol's husband, Bill and their family.

I am so blessed to know so many Christ-filled people. How much He must love me to put all of them into my life and I give Praise, Honor and Glory to Jesus Christ my Savior and Redeemer.

Printed in the United States
152867LV00002B/2/P